ABOUT Face

ABOUT Face

a plastic surgeon's 4-step

nonsurgical program

for younger, beautiful skin

Gregory Bays Brown, M.D.

WITH JANE O'BOYLE

Foreword by Sarah Brown,
Beauty editor, *Vogue*

Ballantine Books

New York

Copyright © 2005 by Gregory Brown, M.D.

Published in the United States by Ballantine Books, an imprint of The Random
House Publishing Group, a division of Random House, Inc., New York.

Ballantine and colophon are registered trademarks
of Random House, Inc.

Line drawings by Megan O'Boyle on pages 4, 123, and 171
copyright © 2005 by Megan O'Boyle

Grateful acknowledgment is made to Ballantine Books for permission to
reprint excerpts from *20-Minute Yoga Workouts* by the American Yoga
Association, copyright © 1995 by the American Yoga Association and the
Philp Lief Group, Inc. Used by permission of Ballantine Books,
a division of Random House, Inc.

Library of Congress Cataloging-in-Publication Data is available.

ISBN 0-345-46728-0

Printed in the United States of America on acid-free paper

Ballantine Books website address: www.ballantinebooks.com

10 9 8 7 6 5 4 3 2 1

First Edition

Book design by Cassandra J. Pappas

to my partner,

Scott Rogers

acknowledgments

Lynn Rice, Harriet Weintraub, Virginia Coleman, Ralph Akyuz, Susan Goldsberry, Diane Ernst, Summer Thompson, Joshua Houlette, Kathleen Tomarken, Tony Pinho, Robert D. Fields, M.D., Stanley Cohen, Ph.D., Danielle Martin (in memoriam), William Rutter, Ph.D., Maurice Jurkiewicz, M.D., John Bostwick, M.D. (in memoriam), Hazel Wyatt, John Stabenau, Burton M. Tansky, Kate Oldham, Wendy Browning, M. Ronald Ruskin, Karen Arnett Hale, Julee Herdt, Michelle Burke, George King, Carl Riebel, and Harry and Jean Brown.

contents

foreword

Sarah Brown
Beauty editor, Vogue

Why would a plastic surgeon ever—ever!—suggest anything but surgery as a solution to aging skin? Doesn't sound like the most sound business plan, but then again, times are changing. First, a little history:

Once, not long ago, plastic surgeons performed surgery and dermatologists tended to matters of the skin. The lines were clear: Dermatologists specialized in spotting suspicious moles, curing acne, and treating the odd rash, among other things; cosmetic surgeons were the go-to guys (and girls) for nose jobs, liposuction, and the ultimate act of age defiance, the *we're-getting-serious-now* midlife milestone known as the face-lift. The surgery was significant; the results were, in many cases, radical.

The landscape has changed. In the last decade or so, we have become an increasingly youth-obsessed society, seduced by the promise and possibility of halting age in its tracks. More Americans than ever—women and men, young and old—are flocking to medispas and dermatology and plastic surgery offices for line-erasing Botox, collagen, and Restylane injections, complexion-refining chemical peels, and laser treatments. If trainers were the shrinks of the nineties, skin doctors are the gurus of the new millennium.

Which brings up a key point: Somewhere along the line, as the fields of plastic surgery and dermatology evolved to address the growing youth-quake, the two disciplines converged. Though plastic surgeons still keep their scalpels sharp, they've realized that redraping slack skin over muscle is only half the battle. Simply put, the best way to create youthful skin is quite literally *to create youthful skin.* Instead of ironing it out and pulling it tight (the nitty-gritty behind surgery), the focus has shifted to improving the quality of the skin itself, treating it from the inside out by stimulating collagen production and encouraging new cell growth. The fight against age is being fought at the molecular level, and skin care informed by the most sophisticated science is leading the charge.

Dr. Greg Brown, a Louisville, Kentucky, plastic surgeon, was among the first to see the big picture. Understanding the limitations of physical surgery, he looked beyond the boundaries of his discipline to consider the most basic inner workings of the skin: how it behaved under ordinary and extraordinary circumstances, how it repaired and rejuvenated itself, and how it could be manipulated to effect tangible change. The groundbreaking research he helped to pioneer in the early nineties introduced words like *biotechnology* into the cosmetic vernacular and set the stage for a new generation of skin care based on cutting-edge medical discovery.

So are face-lifts a complete relic of the past, and what exactly does this mean for plastic surgeons who are, after all, trained to cut and drape and sew? The most enlightened are evolving their practices to include the latest technology, replacing many of the aggressive, invasive overhauls they might have once recommended with sequences of smaller, more conservative in-office treatments. These mini-procedures, designed to complement daily topical regimens, are "layered" to create cumulative, and therefore more subtle, results. The focus has largely shifted to influencing the way skin behaves, rather than simply operating on it in an effort to smooth things over. And this is good news! If you could avoid sliding under the knife—it's expensive; it's painful; there are risks involved; you have to wear dark glasses and lie to your friends about going on "vacation"—wouldn't you?

This book is designed as a comprehensive guide for navigating the often overwhelming sea of promising new skin care options and for creating a strategic game plan for looking your best at every stage of your life. With science advancing at the speed of light—a newer, better laser or injectible filler introduced every several months, it seems—there are more possibilities than ever. And it's exciting . . . inspiring . . . empowering. Looking younger, brighter, better, is now more attainable than ever—if you play by the rules of the game, which means making healthy lifestyle choices and sticking to them.

When it comes down to it, the true look of youth is less about being ageless (a scary proposition in itself that never quite works out) and more about a complexion distinguished by freshness, radiance, resilience, and evenness of tone—whatever your age. Rather than having the airbrushed (and in turn artificial) look of perceived perfection, it's about a face with luminosity, three-dimensional contours, and natural volume. Consider this your handbook for getting there.

introduction

It has been twenty years since I completed my residency at Massachusetts General Hospital and embarked on the specialty of plastic surgery. In that relatively short time, I have seen aesthetic procedures transformed from standard surgery to innovations using lasers, laparoscopy, and microscopic injections. At the same time, thousands of topical products have appeared, promising to turn back time and erase all signs of aging from your face. Times have changed.

It was only about eighty years ago that it became acceptable for women to simply have their hair styled or their nails manicured at beauty salons. In the first half of the twentieth century, new advances in cosmetics and in advertising appealed to women from all walks of life—suddenly, a waitress could have the same beautiful hairstyle as a society matron. Cosmetic enhancements were seen as a means toward self-empowerment, a sign of self-respect, for all classes of women. It brought about a sense of equality among women, particularly for "aged women"—in the

1930s that meant those over the age of thirty-five! If you could not change social norms about aging then you could, at least, change your appearance to meet the popular standards.

In recent decades, innumerable clinical studies and tests have been performed to prevent or reverse the signs of aging. When it came to improving the life cycle of the human skin cell, however, it seemed little could be done to improve on nature's course, which was the predictable death of the skin cell and its slowed renewal. Until the 1980s, skin care had not changed in thousands of years. Milk baths, mineral oil, and lanolin were still used for the same purposes as they were in the days of Cleopatra. In other words, the only thing we could do to optimize the condition of our skin was to use a moisturizer. As recently as 1980, researchers had accepted the idea that they could not even hasten the natural human process of healing injured skin. Doctors knew that they should keep a wound moist and free from infection, but were not aware of any additional treatment that would actually accelerate the healing. As I worked with burn victims and surgical patients in my residency and practice, I was determined to find out how skin really worked, and what could affect the way it regenerated itself.

As a plastic surgeon, I have spent years observing the process of how skin heals. In clinical studies, I innovated the application of a human protein that actually makes skin heal faster than its usual rate, a landmark discovery that was originally published in the *New England Journal of Medicine*. Medical scientists had long believed that nothing could be done to accelerate skin regeneration in normal patients, under optimal conditions, but these clinical studies proved otherwise. After several years of research, my tests began to prove what some had thought was impossible—that the quality of normal skin growth could be altered with a topical treatment. At the same time, I observed that this faster cell growth greatly improved the overall condition and appearance of skin; even skin that was not injured was rejuvenated.

I began to focus on applying this human protein to skin that was not wounded or burned, but simply aging normally. The results were astounding. Middle-aged skin cells replaced themselves as quickly as a youngster's skin cells. The protein is called Epidermal Growth Factor (EGF). It manipulates skin cell growth at the molecular level—creating firm new skin as quickly as a teenager's body does, no matter your age.

In the last five years, my colleagues and I have developed topical products containing EGF as well as proteins in the form of two other human growth factors. They are the first skin care products that contain the protein of human cells, produced through bioengineering, rather than those derived from plants or animals. Only human proteins can really interact effectively with human skin. The more I learned about new levels of technology that could lead to innovative applications in skin care, the more I realized that consumers should be made aware of these new developments as quickly as possible. I compiled data not only from my own research, but from laboratories around the world. I wrote this book to delineate the facts and fallacies of skin products, and to inform readers about what they can do now, and what products they can look forward to using in the coming years. If you were considering having a cosmetic procedure, this book may prompt you to reconsider your options.

People are living longer than ever before, and most are now aware that a healthy lifestyle enhances the quality of everything they do. Millions of people have learned how to take care of their bodies and to maintain good health with proper exercise and diet. Yet that same awareness generally does not exist for the enhancement and vitality of the largest human organ: the skin.

Bones and muscles directly respond to diet and exercise, but not so easily the lines and wrinkles on your face and neck.

Even with today's skin care advances, we are only in the very early stages of a medical revolution. It's an exciting time for a doctor like me who specializes in skin treatments and cosmetic surgery. In the next twenty-five years, we are going to see biotechnology such as recombinant DNA and stem cell and gene therapies change the face of skin care as we know it. I am sure that one day simple creams will supplant the need for cosmetic surgery. Until then, however, the consumer is being bombarded with "new" skin care products at breakneck speed, most of which are nothing more than moisturizers or sunscreens behind colorful advertising and promotion. My goal with this book is to bring you up to date on the current technological innovations for effective skin care, and to inform you about new treatments that are still in the test stages but will soon be available to help you rejuvenate and maintain more beautiful skin.

In addition to my research, another factor influenced my pursuit of nonsurgical antiaging technologies. As a plastic surgeon, I know it is possible to re-create a youthful appearance with surgery. However, it is not possible to use surgical means to re-create youth itself—truly younger skin can be achieved only at the molecular level. No matter how superb the surgeon's skills are, the results of a face-lift are often disappointing to the consumer: Instead of restored youth, you might simply have a "surgerized" result. This is often not appealing. There is no surgical way to achieve the wonderful, fluid-filled undereye tissue of an eighteen-year-old. But that look can now be achieved through bioengineered skin treatments at the molecular level. Surgery is rejuvenation on a "macro level," whereas molecular engineering brings on "micro level" changes.

My four-step skin care program begins with systemic care—treating your whole body with proper nutrients is essential to good skin. The first two steps are diet and exercise routines that bring out the best in your skin. Think of these as skin care from the inside out. I then prescribe a daily regimen of cleansing, toning, and protection, explaining how each affects the replenishment of new skin. The final step of my program is a customized noninvasive treatment, depending on your needs and goals. Some of these treatments are not yet on the market, but I include them here in Part Two, to fully inform you so you can prepare for your future needs.

A friend of mine, fifty-nine-year-old Sheila P., has had three face-lifts over the past two decades. She tells me that, had she known about topical treatments that are now available, she probably would not have opted for surgery at all. More and more of my patients are choosing nonsurgical options. In 2003, nearly 9 million people consulted a doctor about improving their appearance, and fewer than 1.8 million had actual surgery. Most patients chose a nonsurgical option, such as a chemical peel, microdermabrasion, or an injection of Botox or collagen. Every day, the nonsurgical options are becoming even more intensive and varied. There will be many more within the next ten years.

Genetic modification has brought us to a point where you can buy a houseplant that has never grown in nature. A mutant fish has been created to glow in the dark, to identify water pollution. Now you can buy that fish for your home aquarium. The human appetite for altering nature—including the human body—will lead us to the day when gene-filled injections allow an individual to choose the color of his skin or hair, body type, even how and when she will grow old. We're not there yet, but we are on our way. You need to know what will be possible in the years to come.

With this book, you can map out an immediate plan, and also a lifetime plan for aesthetic skin care and skin treatments.

I am a plastic surgeon, yet I know that surgery will eventually be less and less important for major aesthetic improvements, perhaps even within my lifetime. Unlike many plastic surgeons, I dedicate my practice to the least invasive treatment possible for the desired result. Unlike dermatologists, I understand what can and cannot be accomplished with surgical intervention. The third section of this book focuses on the optimal procedures for patients in particular age groups. I encourage you to read the whole book, no matter your age. You will learn things about the evolution of your complexion that will help you now and in the future. I also encourage you to read this book even if you have already had a face-lift. All of the new options can help anyone look better, regardless of how you have cared for your skin in the past. The second section provides you with examples of the treatment options you have now, and previews innovative new techniques that will soon be available to you. After reading this book, you might discuss parts of it with your plastic surgeon or dermatologist to determine the best course of action for you.

I firmly believe that the true source of beauty is not always lifts, nips, or tucks. It is the newly discovered ability of your skin to regain the glow of youth. Educating yourself about this technology is the best treatment money can buy. This book will affect how you care for your skin, for the rest of your life.

ABOUT Face

how skin works

The skin is the largest organ of the body. It is about two one-hundredths of an inch thick, and covers an area of roughly twenty square feet. Its inner layers are called the *dermis,* which contains blood vessels and cells known as fibroblasts. These cells produce collagen, elastin, and proteoglycans, the mortar that holds your skin together. The outer component is the *epidermis.* This contains somewhere between twelve and fifteen layers of cells but, as we age, they diminish to nine or ten layers. Only the very bottom layers of cells divide and replace themselves. They slowly rise to the skin's surface and, as they rise, the cells lose their nuclei and die. This outer layer—known as the *stratum corneum*—is then imperceptibly sloughed off in tiny pieces during everyday activity, which in turn compels the bottom layer to start making new skin cells. In a teenager this exfoliation cycle takes about two or three weeks; if your skin is injured, the process goes into overdrive to make new skin to replace the damaged.

This replacement cycle slows with aging, as the cells become sluggish, less apt to divide, and less hydrated.

Part of this cycle is affected by the formation of free radicals. These are oxygen molecules that have an odd number of electrons, causing them to be unstable. As they seek out healthier electrons from other molecules, including those of our skin cells, free radicals cause a chain reaction of damage known as *oxidation*. Free radicals not only harm skin cells, but they are known to impede blood circulation and cause varicose veins. The most significant external sources of free radicals are cigarette smoke, air pollution, and pesticides.

The growing susceptibility to free radicals is one of the causes of aging in various parts of our bodies. Antioxidants such as vitamin C and vitamin E have been shown to defend against free radicals, lending the free radicals their own electrons and forming a

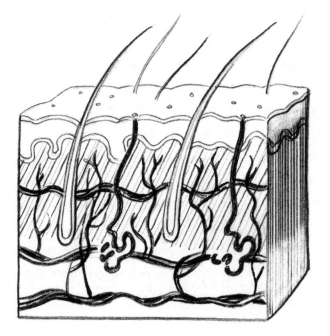

barrier that protects human skin cells. These vitamins are found in a variety of vegetables, meat, and dairy products.

The cycle is also affected by a number of other factors, such as diet, sun exposure, smoking, and physical exercise. No doubt, you already know that some of these behaviors and habits are harmful to your body. Let me tell you how they specifically affect your skin.

Your Face Is a Reflection of How You Eat

The average American's diet is filled with carbohydrates, sugar, salt, and caffeine. If you kept track of these elements over the course of just one day, you would be amazed at the quantity you consume. Of all of these, sugar and carbohydrates have the worst effects on your complexion. They cause inflammation of the epidermis, and rob your skin of the oxygen it needs to stay youthful. On the other hand, there are foods that feed your skin helpful nutrients and oxygen, such as fish, walnuts, and olive oil. You cannot improve your skin without first addressing your daily diet, which is detailed in Chapter 2. In only a week, you will see clearer skin and feel the effects of rejuvenated oxygen flow throughout your body.

Smoking

This habit creates a toxic metabolism in your whole body. Many people know the lungs are damaged by smoking, which is harmful enough in itself. The more visible effects are in oxygen-deprived skin. When you smoke, it shows on your face. In addition to more wrinkles around the lips and eyes, smokers have skin that is slower to heal. Blood is actually directed away from the skin by the destructive effects of nicotine, causing a grayish tone. We call this overall effect "smoker's skin." The physiological basis is that nicotine causes the tiny subdermal capillaries to go into chronic spasms. These capillaries are the only source of blood supply to your skin. Over time, such decreased oxygen causes the skin to age more rapidly.

Many doctors, including myself, will not perform a cosmetic procedure on someone who smokes. Healing takes longer and the results will be minimized. I will prescribe the patch or nicotine gum or whatever it takes to help a patient quit smoking, and I will permit cosmetic procedures three weeks after that patient has stopped smoking.

A fifty-year-old patient, Robert Z., was scheduled to have a complete face-lift. In order to do it, he finally stopped smoking after twenty-one years. After two months, he saw extreme improvement in his complexion, and in the definition of his cheeks and chin. He looked so good—just from quitting smoking—that all he needed was a medium peel to smooth out his skin tone. He looks years younger and spent a small fraction of the money he'd planned to spend on surgery. Even better: He still doesn't smoke.

Lifestyle

A sedentary life leads to weight gain, which, among many other debilitating effects, simply stretches the skin, even in the face. Stores of fat form cellulite, and sometimes affect blood flow to the hands and feet. Fat also stores testosterone, which can promote adult acne, excessive hair growth, and blotchy skin. Without modest exercise, the entire human body is operating on less oxygen than it was designed for. Bones deteriorate and lose calcium. As with all organs of the body, the skin needs large amounts of oxygen, not only from the outside but from the inside as well. There are fun and simple tricks to getting your body in motion, and Step 2 of my program details exactly how you can incorporate exercise into the busiest schedule.

Sun Exposure

The sun is 93 million miles away, but it is your skin's worst enemy. Some experts say that you accumulate a lifetime of skin damage from the sun by the time you turn eighteen. While I agree that the early years of sun exposure can cause skin cancer decades later, I also believe that sun exposure in your later years is equally damaging. I always insist my patients use sunscreen, regardless of their age, skin type, or outdoor activity. Poor diet, smoking, and air pollution may take their toll, but the sun causes 90 percent of the damage to your skin. The sun makes your melanin work overtime, darkening your skin pigment to protect it from the sun. When melanocytes behave abnormally, these become "age spots," also known as liver spots or sun spots, in a process doctors call "photoaging." These spots are incapable of fading on their own. They will get worse—even cancerous—if you don't act to prevent sun exposure. All of my topical recommendations in Step 3 require the use of sunscreen.

Genetics

Heredity plays a huge role in how our skin ages. How we age is encoded into our individual DNA, largely determining our personal biological clock no matter our skin care habits. The good news is this: My research and that of others have proved that bioengineered products can alter the inherited behavior of our skin. Even more significant, we can change our inherited skin characteristics by eating better, getting exercise, and properly caring for and protecting our skin. We can also choose a special noninvasive procedure, outlined in Step 4, to counteract skin traits that we inherited.

Four Steps to Fabulous Skin

The first two steps of my program condition your skin from the inside out. Many people underestimate the fact that, in order to have youthful skin, they must keep their internal machine operating at optimum condition. Oxygen-rich blood flow, nutrients, and most essential vitamins feed your skin from the deepest layers. If they are not in good condition, your skin will never improve.

The third and fourth steps treat the surface of the skin, literally changing its gene-encoded behavior. These steps are not identical for every person. You know this already, perhaps, if you've tried your friend's favorite skin cream (which did nothing for you) or raced out for the newest filler injection, only to find it faded away after a couple of days. Every person's face is a unique combination of skin, muscle, eyes, mouth, nose, lips, emotional expression, and shield against environment. We are born with incredibly complex features—who needs the perfect nose or voluptuous lips? I don't want my patients to have their friends remark, "Have you had a face-lift?" I want them to say, "You look great!" The goal of my program is to bring your face vibrancy and glowing beauty, and to provide you with the peace of mind and self-assurance that comes from knowing that you look incredible.

Before you begin the four-step program, see how you rate when it comes to the essentials of skin care.

Do you smoke?

    1. never

    2. rarely

    3. frequently

Do you eat a lot of sugars and carbohydrates?

    1. never

    2. rarely

    3. frequently

How much time each day do you spend outdoors?

    1. Only a few minutes, going in and out of the car and shopping

    2. Only when I work in the garden or jog

    3. Every chance I get

Do you get any exercise?

    1. Daily

    2. Twice a week, on average

    3. Twice a month, on average

Is there a history of skin cancer in your family?

    1. No

    2. I don't know

    3. Yes

When you were young, did you spend a lot of time in the sun?

1. Never

2. Rarely

3. Yes

Do you visit a dermatologist?

1. Yes, every year

2. Only when I have a specific problem

3. Never

Do you use sunscreen?

1. Every day

2. When I remember it

3. Only when I'm outdoors

Add up the numbers before your answers. If your total score is between 8 and 12, you have a head start on the transformation of your complexion. If you scored between 13 and 16, you have a few marks against you, but you will compensate for these in only a few days of my program. If you scored between 17 and 24, you have a greater risk of health problems. However, you can completely turn this around in just four weeks on my program. And you, more than the others, will see the most improvements in that short time. Much of the damage may already be done—but, incredibly, much of it can also be reversed.

PART 1

the 4-step program

CHAPTER 2

step 1: eat right—systemic skin care for the whole body

Years ago, my mother believed (or at least she used to tell me) that eating french fries caused acne. Maybe where you come from it was chocolate. While this isn't precisely true, there is no doubt that your eating habits largely contribute to the health of your skin, as much as or even more than they affect the rest of your body.

I don't prescribe an actual diet for my patients, but the low-glycemic-index focus of the Sugar Busters! diet is very good for your complexion and overall health. Learning which foods are good for you, as well as which ones should be avoided, can help you to modify your eating habits without feeling as if you are being deprived or supervised. I provide patients with a simple list of foods that are best for the health of your skin. The foods on this list bring more oxygen to your skin and reduce the harmful effects of sugar. Sugar binds to your body's enzymes and slows them down. Enzymes are the hardworking molecules that facilitate the trillions of your body's chemical reactions on a normal day. This diet keeps your enzymes sleek and agile, and it also might help you to lose weight. I have kept my list simple so you can easily remember it and adhere to it. I don't provide portion restrictions, because I don't consider this a weight-loss diet. This is an antiaging diet. Your body will know how many calories it needs to maintain its vitality.

Dr. Brown's Diet for Glowing Skin

PROTEIN

Eggs

Chicken

Turkey

Fish

Skim or low-fat milk

Soy milk

CARBOHYDRATES

Rolled oats

Whole grain bread, no more than two slices per day

All vegetables, particularly green ones such as broccoli,
spinach, lettuce, and asparagus

Tomatoes

Apples

Berries

All citrus fruits

HEALTHFUL FATS

Olives

Olive oil

Flaxseed oil

Omega fish oils

Unsalted nuts

If you eat primarily the foods on this list, you can have spectacular skin and a well-balanced diet. Adding dashes of lemon, garlic, pepper, cumin, herbs, and other spices will offer variety, and you'll find most restaurants offer delightful variations of these foods. Just don't eat the bread, and don't eat dessert! Both are loaded with sugars. My personal mantra is this: if the food is white (such as potatoes, rice, sugar, pasta), it's probably not good for my body. There is a good sugar substitute called Splenda, which you can use if you must have sweets. Herbal tea is always preferable to caffeine, but coffee is not nearly as toxic as sugar.

Every day, try to eat only foods from this list. You will begin to remember and even to physically sense the foods that are healthy for you. If you stray and eat rice now and then, or a piece of birthday cake, that's okay. My idea of a diet allows you to eat these things on occasion, as long as you return to the list at your next meal. Your body will lead you back to the healthy diet, which will become more and more instinctive as your body reacts with buoyant energy levels, brighter moods, and clearer skin.

This is basically a low-glycemic-index diet. The glycemic index of a food is the measure of how rapidly sugar, or glucose, is absorbed into the bloodstream and raises your natural insulin levels. High insulin levels and repeated "spikes" of insulin from sugar cause more aging than foods with a low glycemic index. Simple carbs such as potatoes and pasta go almost directly into the bloodstream—you feel their effects immediately. That is why such things are known as "comfort food." But these high levels of insulin cause enzymes to get bound and sluggish from sugar.

Imagine pulling a nylon rope across a carpet. Now, imagine wrapping the rope with Velcro first and then pulling it across a carpet. It is nearly impossible to move. This is how glycating sugars affect your enzymes, which control all of the constant changes in your body, including how you age.

I think it is unrealistic to expect a patient to eat salmon twice a day and swallow twenty-five vitamin supplement tablets. A simple, low-glycemic-index diet will enhance your complexion and be easy to adopt for a lifetime, not just for a month or two. *All things in moderation.* Medical studies have proved that restriction of calories (while maintaining nutrients and vitamins) significantly slows the overall aging process by reducing the damage caused by free radical molecules. Some researchers have pointed to the population of Okinawa, Japan, as an example of this theory. Residents there have traditionally consumed a low-calorie diet. As a result, they are forty times more likely than Americans to reach the age of one hundred years.

What Not to Eat

Just as there is a good foods list, there is a bad foods list. Each of these foods contains excessive sugars, which are harmful to healthy skin. As I said earlier, I have a personal rule of thumb: Most food that is white—e.g., pasta, rice, potatoes, bread—is to be avoided. Others include cookies, candy, cakes, muffins, and whole milk.

Vitamin Supplements

It's very difficult to prove the effects of any of the expensive, unregulated supplements currently sold at pharmacies and health food stores. This multibillion-dollar industry is actually a sort of wild and woolly uncontrolled clinical trial where the consuming public is acting as a collective guinea pig. Most researchers still believe the most effective source of vitamins is a balanced diet low in sugar, in which the vitamins are provided in their natural form and not in supplements. My diet satisfies your body's needs for vitamins and minerals. In fact, when someone is planning aesthetic surgery, I instruct the patient to cease using vitamin supplements in the weeks before surgery, as some can cause excessive bleeding. For other people, however, I do recommend taking a daily multivitamin supplement, simply as a precautionary action. It's important to ensure that your body is getting complete replenishment of calcium, vitamin B, and vitamin D. A regular multivitamin does this quite well. Most readily available brands are perfectly acceptable: One A Day, Centrum, even generic brands. No additional pills, in any magic combination or quantity, are truly essential for a healthy body and healthy skin. Keep it simple.

Certain vitamin and herbal supplements are associated with maintaining youth, vigor, and healthy skin. Although these are not established claims, you may check the list of ingredients in your vitamins for the following elements, which are frequently mentioned as barriers to the overall effects of aging.

Antiaging Supplement	Research Reveals	Other Claims	Possible Side Effects of Overuse
Vitamin A (retinol)	Antioxidant; needed for vision, bone development, reproduction, immune function; used for acne	Enhances learning, memory, immune system function; helps prevent dry skin	Headache, fatigue, joint pain, GI distress, hair loss

Natural sources for vitamin A are primarily found in squashes, cayenne pepper, parsley, spinach, broccoli, sweet potatoes, lettuce, tomatoes, and melons. Vitamin A is also found in carrots and beets, and liver. Eating one serving of spinach provides you with all the vitamin A you need for a whole day.

Vitamin C (ascorbic acid)	Antioxidant; needed for growth and repair of connective tissue, bone, teeth	Protects against cancer; enhances immune system function; helps vision problems; slows cellular aging; helps production of collagen; fights stress; promotes wound healing	Increased iron absorption

Vitamin C is found in citrus fruits, tomatoes, berries, apples, broccoli, green leafy vegetables, bell peppers, and hot peppers.

Vitamin E (tocopherol)	Antioxidant; decreases angina and coronary risk; improves skin	Protects against cancer; enhances immune system function; helps vision problems; slows cellular aging	May decrease the antioxidants that protect against nitrogen oxides

Natural sources of vitamin E include whole grains, eggs, olives, parsley, nuts, and green leafy vegetables.

Selenium	Antioxidant; deficiency linked to cancer and heart disease	Protects against cancer and AIDS-related illnesses	Irritability, fatigue, nerve damage, GI upset
Chromium	Intensifies insulin; deficiency linked to	Increases strength and lean body	Iron deficiency, skin problems,

	adult-onset diabetes; most Americans are deficient	mass; stabilizes blood sugars; lowers cholesterol levels	increased risk of lung cancer
Coenzyme Q10	Antioxidant; protects against reperfusion damage, congestive heart failure, muscular dystrophy	Enhances sports performance; protects against cancer and gum disease	
Garlic	Improves lipid profile; protects against cardiovascular disease	Protects against cancer	
Ginkgo	Treats dementia, depression, and concentration deficits		GI upset
Ginseng	Prevents colds and flu	Improves mood	Hypoglycemia, insomnia, diarrhea
Grape seed	Antioxidant	Improves circulation, slows macular degeneration, myopia	Liver toxicity (in animals)

Some believe that it is the grape seed that lends red wine its medicinal qualities for coronary health.

Although I do not believe multiple supplements are necessary, I am intrigued by a new product called Olivenol, a pill derived from the water in olives. The patented extraction is called Hidrox, or hydroxytyrosol. Ounce per ounce, hydroxytyrosol contains more antioxidants than vitamin C, grape-seed oil, and green tea combined. Some experts credit a diet containing olive oil with improving moisture in the skin, lowering bad cholesterol, and preventing cancer and coronary heart disease. This has been suspected for centuries, particularly by populations in the olive-rich regions surrounding the Mediterranean Sea. A few years ago, there was great acclaim about Oleuropin, the extract of the olive leaf, but that supplement proved to be poorly absorbed into the bloodstream. Not so Olivenol, which is derived from the watery pulp of organic olives. One pill contains the equivalent antioxidant benefits of six ounces of olive oil, and none of the fat. Olivenol can be purchased at vitamin retail outlets as well as online through sites such as GetVitamins.com, MotherNature.com, and OutletNutrition.com.

Of course, olive oil is included in my list of good foods to eat. Extra virgin olive oil contains the most nutrients. Add just a little olive oil on a salad or a grilled vegetable, and you don't need to take any supplements. But it is intriguing to see how science continues to improve on the uses of ancient remedies.

Liquids

All doctors will tell you that drinking water brings huge benefits to your body, largely because it is a great infusion of oxygen, carrying power to all parts of your body. You should drink at least six glasses of water every day.

A high consumption of alcohol is never good for you. Alcohol can promote the onset of rosacea, which appears as chronic redness in the face. Alcohol can also cause adult acne and rhinophyma, the condition where capillaries in the nose are broken and sometimes inflamed. Picture the nose of W. C. Fields, and you know what rhinophyma looks like. Most of us are not excessive drinkers. But even a single scotch or vodka—or any distilled spirits—contains vast amounts of carbohydrates and sugar, as do beer and wine. However, some studies have shown that a modest consumption of red wine can serve as a tonic to the cardiovascular system, and can stimulate the production of HDL, the so-called good cholesterol. These studies have indicated that one or two glasses of red wine per day—and no more—may be a healthy source of antioxidants.

If you're at a party or restaurant and the fattening appetizers are tempting you, treat yourself to a glass of good red wine instead.

A Sample Menu of Options for Skin Health and Vitality

These suggestions will give you a good idea of how easy it is to adapt to a wide variety of healthy foods in your everyday life. You can choose from the foods listed here and create a balanced meal.

BREAKFAST (WITH COFFEE OR TEA)
> Orange or grapefruit, whole fruit or as juice
> Strawberries or blueberries
> Skim milk
> 2 eggs, or
> 1 serving of oatmeal (unflavored); sprinkle with Splenda, if
>   desired, or
> Whole grain Cheerios, puffed kashi, shredded wheat, or bran
> Whole grain toast
> Buckwheat pancakes with sugar-free jam

LUNCH (DRINK WATER OR TEA)
> Turkey sandwich on whole grain bread, such as whole wheat,
>   whole rye, or pumpernickel

Lean roast beef or ham and cheese sandwich on whole grain bread (add light mayonnaise, mustard, tomato, and lettuce, if desired)

Canned tuna with chopped celery

Cheeseburger on whole grain bun

Peanut butter and sugar-free jelly on whole grain bread

Chicken salad on lettuce with whole grain toast

Cobb salad (julienned turkey, ham, and Swiss cheese with hard-boiled egg) with sugar-free dressing and one slice pumpernickel toast

Grilled skinless chicken Caesar salad

Pickle or olives

Celery sticks

DINNER (SERVED WITH WATER OR TEA)

Grilled pork tenderloin or veal chop

Broiled salmon with lemon juice and dill

Grilled tuna or other fish

Grilled chicken with olive oil, onion, and celery

Grilled lean sirloin or New York strip steak

Grilled lamb patty

Ground beef cooked with sugar-free tomato sauce

Baked turkey breast rubbed with salt, pepper, and thyme

Skinless chicken, baked or grilled with spices

Grilled eggplant slices

Steamed green beans, asparagus, or broccoli

Steamed peppers and garlic or cauliflower

Baked onions

Broiled tomato with basil

Mushrooms sautéed in olive oil

Baby lima beans, snow peas, or spicy black-eyed peas

Cooked spinach

Pea soup

Green salad with tomato, artichoke hearts, blue cheese, pine
nuts, oil, and vinegar

Brown rice

Whole wheat pasta sprinkled with olive oil and Romano
cheese

SNACKS (2 PER DAY)

1 apple, peach, or orange

1 pear or slice of melon

Low-fat cottage cheese

Berries

12 nuts or grapes

3 whole grain crackers

Sugar-free frozen yogurt

2 small pieces of cheese

Drugs

As Americans age, they are consuming more and more prescription drugs, many of which have damaging effects on the skin. There are also hormone supplements and birth control medications that affect the condition of skin. If you notice unusual changes in your complexion, notify your doctor. The reaction in your skin may reflect a more severe reaction taking place in your system. Every body is different but, frequently, taking an alternative medication will make the side effects disappear.

Here is a partial list of popular prescription supplements that are said to hold off the effects of aging:

Supplement	Used For	Extra Benefits	Side Effects
Dehydroepiandrosterone (DHEA)	Adrenal hormone; deficiency linked to heart disease and breast cancer	Slows aging; prevents or treats Alzheimer's disease; protects against some cancer	Some evidence of certain cancer risks
Estrogen	Improves bone mineral density and lipid profile; promotes vaginal epithelial growth and lubrication	Enhances cognition	Increased risk of breast and other cancers and gallbladder disease; thromboembolism
Testosterone	Improves bone mineral density; stimulates libido; increases red cell mass and strength, decreases adipose tissue		Increased risk of breast and prostate cancer; hepatic toxicity; polycythemia; cardiovascular disease; impotence
Human Growth Hormone	Strengthens bone; improves mental clarity, immune function, skin structure		Hypoglycemia; edema; muscle and joint pain; carpal tunnel syndrome; hypertension; may enhance growth of certain cancers

Marla G., a twenty-four-year-old secretary, came to see me about smoothing out her acne scars. Her skin was in poor condition, but she was also thirty pounds overweight. I gave her my list of skin-healthy foods, and treated her with a medium facial peel. I also prescribed that she go on a thirty-minute walk, five days a week. In addition to the exercising, I recommended that she increase her consumption of water. (If you add eight glasses of water to your daily diet for only one month, you will lose weight even if you don't change other dietary or exercise habits.) *All* of these things gave her complexion a revitalized glow. These effects on the skin are a result of increasing one's basal metabolic rate (the calories required to help your skin every day), which increases muscle-to-fat ratio as well as blood flow to the skin.

If you follow the diet plan above, take a multivitamin every day, and perform moderate exercise, you will have taken the most important step in improving your skin. You will notice the difference in your complexion within one week. In two months, without doing anything other than following this diet, your skin will be years younger. But there are other steps that complement the diet, and that also show on your face.

DR. BROWN'S 7-DAY DIET FOR GLOWING SKIN

Here's a sample of a week's menus that will transform your skin. Be sure to include a multivitamin every day, as well as lots of water.

DAY 1   **Breakfast:** 2 scrambled eggs, blueberries with skim milk, coffee

Lunch: Chicken salad on lettuce, sliced tomato, 5 olives, iced tea

Snack: Frozen yogurt

Dinner: Pea soup, grilled pork chop, sautéed green beans in olive oil and pine nuts, salad with feta cheese, honeydew melon, tea with Splenda

Snack: 2 handfuls of unsalted peanuts

DAY 2   **Breakfast:** Oatmeal with strawberries and skim milk, cantaloupe slice

Snack: 5 whole grain crackers and cheese

Lunch: Cheeseburger on whole grain bun, pickles, tomatoes, coffee

Snack: Low-fat cottage cheese

Dinner: Grilled tuna, black-eyed peas with salsa, sautéed mushrooms, slice of whole grain bread, frozen yogurt

DAY 3   **Breakfast:** Whole wheat waffles with sugar-free jam, coffee, raspberries

Lunch: Tuna sandwich on whole grain bread, small green salad, coffee

Snack: A handful of unsalted nuts, 4–6 olives

Dinner: Grilled chicken with olive oil, onion, celery, sautéed mushrooms and snow peas, hot tea

Snack: Apple

DAY 4   **Breakfast:** Shredded wheat cereal with blueberries and skim milk, coffee

Snack: Orange

Lunch: Ham and cheese sandwich on whole grain bread with lettuce, tomato, and mayonnaise, steamed broccoli

Snack: Cold steamed asparagus with spicy peanut sauce

Dinner: Broiled salmon with lemon and dill, brown rice, sautéed artichoke hearts with sun-dried tomatoes, coffee

Snack: 3 celery sticks with peanut butter

DAY 5   **Breakfast:** Half a grapefruit with Splenda, whole grain toast with sugar-free jam

Lunch: Chef's salad with turkey, cheese, and low-fat dressing, pumpernickel toast, tea

Snack: Cottage cheese and crackers

Dinner: Whole grain pasta with sautéed tomatoes in olive oil and garlic, seared scallops, and spinach salad with blue cheese

Snack: Frozen yogurt

DAY 6   **Breakfast:** Bowl of Cheerios with blueberries, coffee

Snack: One handful of unsalted cashews

Lunch: Turkey sandwich on whole rye toast, with mustard and Swiss cheese, asparagus, yogurt

Snack: Grilled skinless chicken breast

Dinner: Pork tenderloin with apples, baked onions, steamed cauliflower in mustard sauce

DAY 7   **Breakfast:** Buckwheat pancakes with strawberries, coffee

Snack: Pear and blue cheese

Lunch: Open-faced roast beef sandwich, grilled onions, cooked spinach, bowl of berries

Snack: Peach

Dinner: Meat loaf prepared with whole grain bread crumbs, roasted tomatoes, eggplant and asparagus with lemon and garlic, tea

step 2: keep your face in shape by moving your arms and legs

ertain simple routines can greatly improve overall skin health and appearance. For example, practicing yoga has a noticeable effect on skin condition. When you hold a yoga pose for forty or sixty seconds, you are cutting the oxygen supply to designated parts of your body. When you release the pose, blood rushes into these areas, actually increasing the overall blood flow (reactive hyperemia), over and above the normal amounts. You can watch how your skin turns pink with added blood after you release a yoga pose. Over time, this routine will train a constant increased blood flow to these parts, even when you're not doing yoga. This has amazing benefits for your skin, because vessels get narrower as we age, contributing to diabetes, osteoporosis, and oxygen-deprived skin. After all, healthy skin needs oxygen replenishment not just from the outside, but from internal blood flow as well. Yoga helps to increase normal blood flow to all the body's organs, including the skin. Look at people who have practiced yoga for years—Madonna and Sting, for example, have great skin. My yoga instructor is nearing sixty years old, but she looks twenty years younger, and she wears hardly any makeup.

I believe a healthy lifestyle is a matter of having the right attitude—don't do anything that will be difficult to maintain. All things in moderation. Curb your high-reaching goals and just try to do something active at least three times a week. Don't make yourself feel guilty if you take a day or two off. Don't spend a lot of money on a health club or a treadmill if you can't afford it. Who needs that added stress and guilt associated with exercise? One of the best things you can do for your body is to go for a simple walk outdoors.

Walking is a cross-patterned activity—you swing your left leg with your right arm and vice versa. This activity is very calming for your brain, yet stimulating and revitalizing for your body. Even if you are well into middle age, start a walking routine. Begin modestly—twenty-minute jaunts through your neighborhood twice a week. You need nothing more than a good pair of walking shoes. You might invite a friend or neighbor to join you. Work your way up to forty-five minutes, adding speed or hills to the route. One of my patients, Janet S., adopted a large dog to accompany her on her daily jaunts. My friend Elaine takes walks while listening to her favorite morning radio program on a portable headset. She doesn't permit herself to the listen to the show unless she is outside walking at the same time. This is one of several little incentives that can help you keep a routine.

Start taking the stairs instead of using the elevator, and park your car farther away from your usual parking spaces. Even a small amount of physical activity does more than bring oxygen to your skin—it also alleviates stress. Worry can add years to your appearance. In addition to the tensions and strain to your body and overall good health, stress can make you repeatedly frown, squint, and flex your nose and chin. After only a few months, these subconscious actions will leave their mark in the form of lines, wrinkles, pimples, or broken capillaries. In your busy day, make an appointment with yourself. Spend a half hour on yourself, doing something you enjoy, but *doing* something. The pounds will melt away, and so will your stress.

A BEGINNER'S WEEKLY SAMPLER OF HEALTHY ACTIVITY

MONDAY	Attend a yoga class
TUESDAY	Lift hand weights at home while watching television
WEDNESDAY	Go for a brisk twenty-minute walk after work
THURSDAY	Practice stretching or yoga at home with a video
FRIDAY	Take a day of rest, or go dancing!
SATURDAY	Go for a long ninety-minute walk with a friend
SUNDAY	Swim for half an hour, or walk back and forth in waist-high water

Breathe

Many of you have read, time and time again, about the benefits of drinking large quantities of water. I have said it myself. What most of you probably don't realize is that the real reason water is so good for you is because it provides much of your body's internal supply of oxygen. Oxygen is vital to human life, of course, but it is also the primary nutrient for your skin. If you practice yoga, you know how transforming breath work can be during your routine. Twenty minutes of yoga can provide your body with the same increased oxygen as a gallon of water. You can perform yoga at home, at work behind a desk, while you travel, or in a class. Here are tips on a superb exercise regimen, from the American Yoga Association. Doing this routine just two or three times a week will condition your body and your face.

(Note: The following pages are excerpted with illustrations from *20-Minute Yoga Workouts* by the American Yoga Association [New York: Ballantine Books, 1995].)

PHYSICAL BENEFITS OF BREATHING PRACTICE

Regular practice of breathing techniques protects the heart and can help to reduce blood pressure, especially in combination with yoga exercises and meditation. It does this by releasing muscle tension in the autonomic nervous system, which controls the contraction and relaxation of smooth muscles such as the heart and blood vessel walls. Breathing also can relieve insomnia, by relaxing the body and reducing the activity of the mind. If you have trouble sleeping, breathing exercises will help you to achieve peaceful, natural sleep without drugs or alcohol. Athletes use breathing exercises to increase strength and endurance and to be sure the muscles get oxygen to replenish stores depleted through exertion.

HELPFUL HINTS

1. Always breathe in and out through your nose (unless you must breathe through your mouth for medical reasons). In other forms of exercise, the forced exhalation through pursed lips helps to expel air more quickly; for a beginner in yoga, the point in breathing exercises is not to move air quickly but to relax, focus, and concentrate the mind. This can be accomplished much better by slowing down the movement of the breath.

If you find that one nostril is blocked and you can't breathe evenly, there is a simple technique for opening it. Make a fist and apply pressure in the armpit of the side that is open (the nerves that govern your left nostril, for instance, are located on the right side of your body) or lie on your side (again, the side that is open) for a few minutes.

2. Focus your attention on the sound of your breath. By closing your throat slightly, you will notice a steamlike sound, not unlike the sound of a shell held up to your ear at the beach. You will feel it at the back of your throat first, instead of through the front of your nostrils, and it will feel cool. Focusing on the sound of the breath is the fastest way to become more concentrated. Closing your eyes also helps. Another aid is wax earplugs, available at any drugstore—the kind that swimmers use. Knead the wax in your hands to soften it, and press it over the ear opening. If you push it too far in, you'll be distracted by all the sounds your body makes—the blood pulsing, joints creaking, and so on. By just covering the ear opening, you'll intensify the sound of the breath so you can concentrate better, and also remove the distraction of outside noises. If you live on a busy street or feel distracted by other activities going on in your home, use the earplugs for your meditation too.

3. Give yourself time to warm up. Yes, there has to be a warm-up period even in breathing. This means that your first breaths will be shorter, and they will gradually lengthen with practice. Start with relatively short breaths and gradually extend the length with each repetition.

4. Breathing is not a competitive sport! Although the idea should be to gradually extend the breath to longer cycles, the goal in this practice is not simply longer breaths for their own sake; instead, try to notice how you feel while you're breathing, and learn how to use the breath to change how you feel and to answer the needs of the body.

5. Find a comfortable seated position. There is nothing more important in breathing exercises than establishing a position that you can hold for several minutes without strain. Ideally, this would be a seated position where your back is straight. If you are limber enough, sit on the floor with your hips elevated on one or more cushions. Sit cross-legged on the edge of the cushions so your pelvis tilts forward slightly and your knees touch the floor (A). If your knees are still elevated even with the cushions, try straddling the cushions (B). You can also do breathing exercises very successfully while sitting on the edge of a bed or chair (C). The same rule applies—hips higher than knees—so you may have to tuck your toes under to find the correct position for breathing. If you have a bad back, or for some other reason can't find a comfortable seated position, you may do your breathing lying down with cushions under your legs to take pressure off your

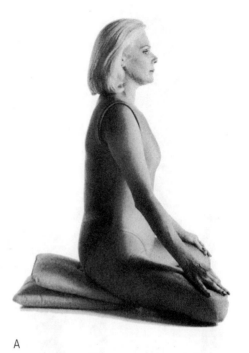

A

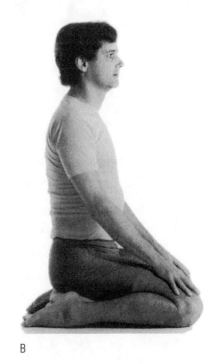

B

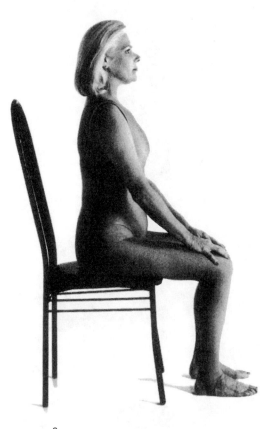

C

lower back. Don't use a pillow under your head; remember, no matter what position you end up in, your spine should remain straight, and that includes the neck. Try not to have any pressure on the back of the head or neck. If your floor is hard, lie on a foam mat or a folded blanket.

The reason it is so important to find the proper position is that when your hips are elevated, your lower back tilts forward slightly and your stomach muscles can relax, allowing you to take fuller, longer, and deeper breaths. If you try to maintain a seated position without a relaxed back and stomach, you won't be able to take a full breath.

6. Keep your arms away from your rib cage. Many people are unsure what to do with their arms and hands. There is no need to hold your hands in any special position. The main point to remember is to keep the rib cage free to expand to its fullest when you breathe in. Put your hands on your knees, on your hips, or on your stomach. Never breathe with your hands in your lap because you won't be able to expand your rib cage completely.

7. Don't hold your breath at any time. Make the transition between inhalation and exhalation, and vice versa, smooth and quiet.

Prana

Prana is a Sanskrit word that is often translated as "breath." For yoga practition-
ers, it has a more subtle meaning—closer to "life." *Prana* means not just the outward manifestation of respiration but the subtle support of breath; in other words,
where breath comes from. Before you feel the breath physically, a signal is sent
from somewhere in your brain to your physical breathing apparatus that says it is
time to breathe. That signal comes from *prana,* the vital life force that flows
throughout the body, affecting its organs and functions in new ways, different from
the way you ordinarily think of your daily functioning. Respiration is only one of the
manifestations of this vital energy. *Prana* can be depleted by depression, a poor
diet, and drugs; it can be replenished by rest, meditation, breathing exercises, and
proper food. Connecting with or increasing *prana* makes you sparkle.

WARM UP

ARM ROLL
*Increases circulation; strengthens back and shoulders; improves range
of motion of shoulders; limbers upper back, chest, and midback muscles.*

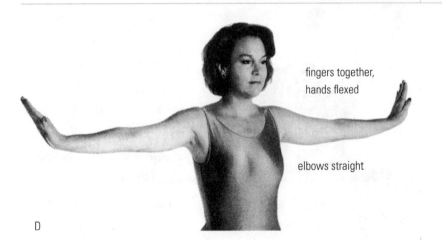

fingers together,
hands flexed

elbows straight

D

Hold your arms straight out to your sides with elbows straight. Face your hands away from you, as if you were stopping traffic on each side of you (D). Holding your arms in this position, slowly rotate them forward in large circles—as large as possible, so you exercise the full range of motion of your shoulder joints. Keep the fingers stretched back. Do 3 or 4 large circles in each direction, then do a few smaller circles in each direction. Let your arms relax, and shake them out.

REPETITIONS: 3–4 in each direction (large circles); 4–5 in each direction (small circles).

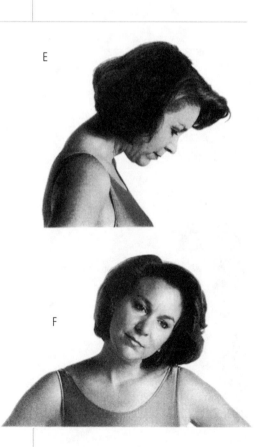

E

F

HEAD ROLL

Limbers neck, spine, and cervical spine; improves circulation in throat.

Stand with arms at your sides or hands on your hips. Keep your shoulders relaxed throughout, breathe normally, and keep your eyes open. Start by bending your head forward and relaxing the back of your neck (E). Slowly rotate your head to one side so your ear is over your shoulder (F). Continue rolling around and tilt your head back carefully (G), then over to the other shoulder, and back to the front. Repeat 3 or more times in each direction. Caution: Do not do this exercise if you have a disk problem in your neck.

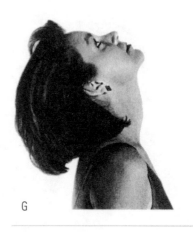

G

REPETITIONS: 3 in each direction.

THIGH STRETCH
Stretches all muscles of the legs and hips; improves respiration.

arch back

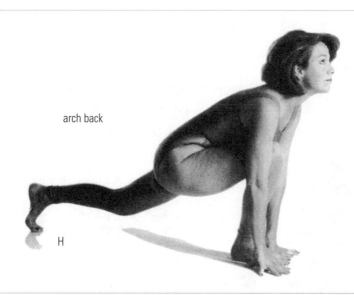

H

Stand with feet a comfortable distance apart and swivel to face right. Bend forward and place your hands on either side of your right foot. Bend your right leg, lower your hips, breathe in, arch your back, and look up (H).

Now breathe out and straighten your legs, tucking your head in toward your right leg (I). Keep the toes of your right foot

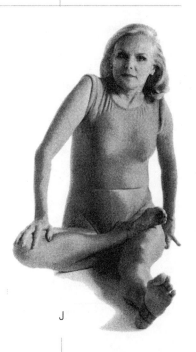

tuck head

straighten legs
as much as
possible

I

toes pointed
forward

pointed. Repeat twice over
the right leg, then stand up
and swivel in the opposite
direction.

REPETITIONS: 3 on each
side.

LIMBER HIPS
Limbers hip and knee joints.

Seated with both legs
stretched in front of you,
carefully lift your right foot
with both hands and place
the ankle on your left thigh. Lean back on
your left hand and press down gently on the
right knee with your right hand (J). Press
and release several times. Use your hands to
carefully lower the leg and switch sides.

REPETITIONS: 5–6 on each side.

KNEE SQUEEZE
*Improves digestion; limbers and relaxes lower
back and hips; improves circulation in pelvic
region.*

Lie on your back with arms over your head
on the floor. Breathe out completely.
Breathe in and lift your left leg and your
head, wrapping your arms around the knee
(K). Hold your breath in and squeeze your

J

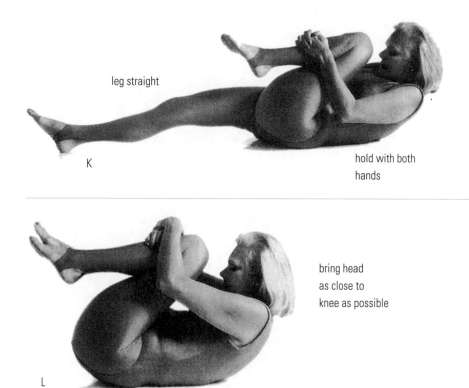

leg straight

K

hold with both
hands

bring head
as close to
knee as possible

L

knee to your chest. Hold for a few seconds, then release, breathe
out, and lower the leg and arm back to the starting position. Repeat with the right leg.

REPETITIONS: 3 on each side.
Now do 3 more repetitions, lifting both legs and your head (L),
with the same breath pattern.

UPPER BODY STRETCH WITH LOCK
*Limbers shoulders and upper back; prevents incontinence; strengthens
lower back and stomach.*

Lie on your back with arms overhead and knees bent. Separate
your feet about 12 inches. Breathe in and stretch your arms and

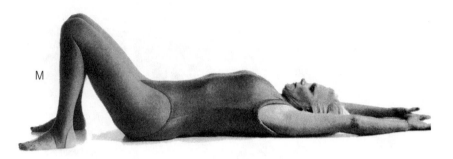

upper torso, then breathe out completely and contract the muscles of your pelvic area (M). Hold for a few seconds, then release.

REPETITIONS: 3

DIAMOND POSE

Sit straight with your knees bent and the soles of your feet touching. Grasp your ankles with both hands and rest your el-

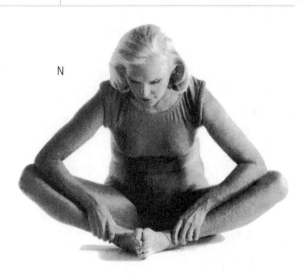

bows on or above your thighs. Breathe in completely, then breathe out as you lean forward slightly and press down on your thighs with your arms (N). Release and repeat twice. Now lace your fingers around your toes, breathe in, and straighten your spine (O). Breathe out as you bend forward, letting your elbows fall outside your legs this time (P). Hold for a few seconds, then breathe in and come back up.

REPETITIONS: 3

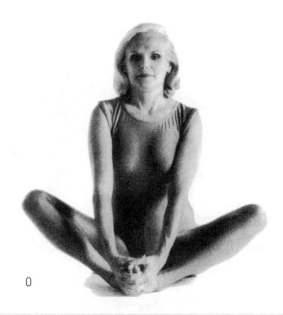

O

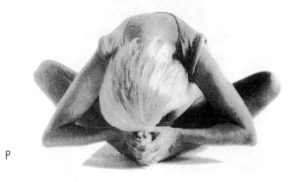

P

CAT BREATH

Limbers lower and midback; tightens stomach muscles; improves breathing.

Start on your hands and knees. Breathe in, arch your back, and look up, so you feel the stretch all along your spine, from tailbone to neck (Q). Then breathe out, round your back, and pull in your stomach to increase the forward stretch (R). Tuck your head.

REPETITIONS: 3

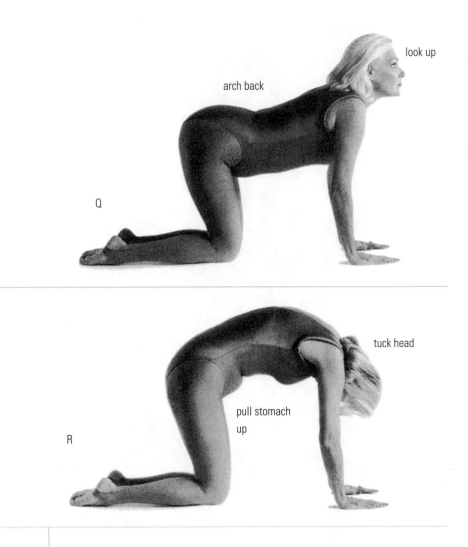

look up

arch back

Q

tuck head

pull stomach up

R

Spine Twist

Improves digestion; limbers and tones entire spine; strengthens and limbers rib cage; relieves chronic constipation; helps relieve bladder, urinary tract, and prostate problems.

Sit with legs outstretched. Bend both knees. Rest your right leg on the floor, and lift your left leg over the right knee; the left foot should be flat (S). Sit up very straight, reach your right arm across your left knee, push the knee as far right as it will go, and grasp the right knee with your right hand; this locks the lower back into position. Your right arm is on the *outside* of your raised (left) leg. Now place your left arm behind you, straighten it, and point the fingers in toward the base of your spine. Look forward, breathe in, then breathe out and twist toward the left as far as possible (T). Look far to the left and stare at one spot. Hold for several seconds, breathing gently. Then release, slowly come forward, and switch sides.

REPETITIONS: 1 on each side

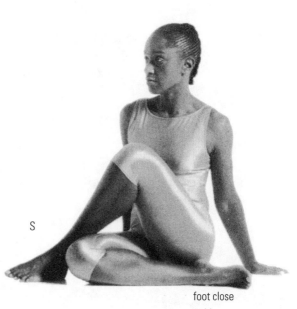

S

foot close
to hip

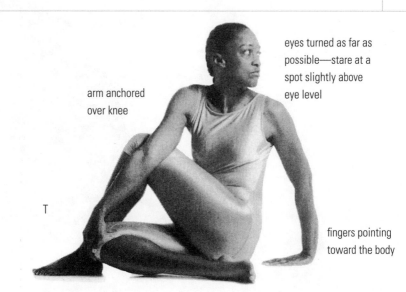

arm anchored
over knee

eyes turned as far as
possible—stare at a
spot slightly above
eye level

T

fingers pointing
toward the body

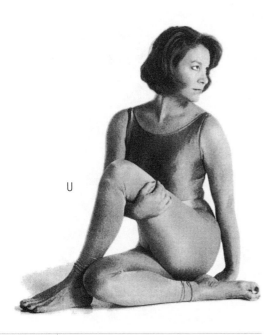

U

After the Spine Twist, stretch both legs out straight and stretch forward over your legs for a few seconds to straighten your spine before going on to the Shoulder Stand.

If your hips and knees are too stiff to do the Spine Twist comfortably, try one of these variations: Instead of crossing the right arm over the left (raised) knee, reach under the knee and grasp the thigh (U). Breathe in completely, breathe out, and twist left as above. Alternatively, you can keep the right leg straight. Twist and breathe as above (V).

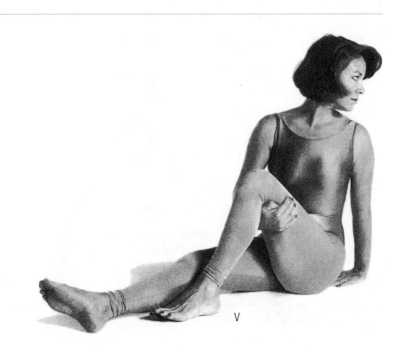

V

SHOULDER STAND

Stimulates thyroid and parathyroid; enhances function of all vital organs; relieves tension on heart and lungs; relaxes nervous system; removes fatigue.

If you have a disk problem in your neck, do not do this exercise or the Plow. Substitute the Easy Bridge (pictured on page 49) instead. This exercise has many benefits. Hold it as long as you can comfortably. Start by sitting with knees drawn up to chest and arms wrapped around knees. Gently roll back and forth a few times to make sure that the spine is in place with no pinched nerves or strained muscles (W). Then roll all the way back, keeping knees to forehead, and immediately support your back with your hands (X). Hold this position until you feel steady, then slowly straighten your legs (Y). If your legs appear to be more at a 45-degree angle, move your hands down your back toward the floor and tuck your chin into your chest; your legs should straighten a bit more. Fix your gaze on the space between your big toes. Relax your breath. Hold as long as you can comfortably.

Go on to the Plow or come out of the pose by bending your

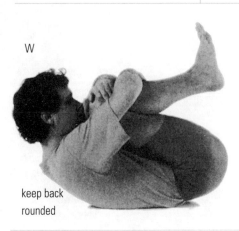

W

keep back
rounded

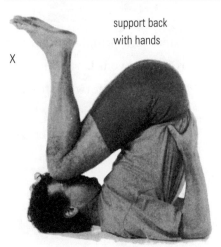

support back
with hands

X

Y

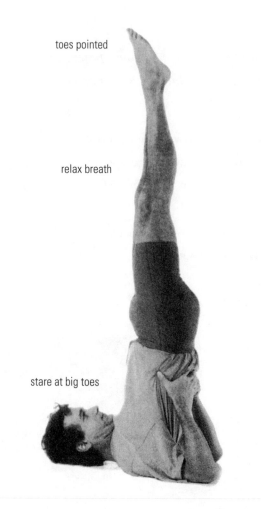

toes pointed

relax breath

stare at big toes

knees and bringing them to your forehead. Slowly roll forward, rounding your back, until you come all the way up to a seated position. Bend forward for a few seconds to be sure the blood doesn't drain from your head too fast.

REPETITIONS: 1

PLOW

Stimulates thyroid; stretches entire spine; reduces body fat; stretches arteries and veins.

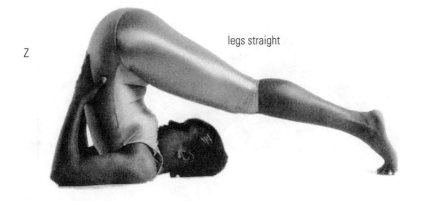

legs straight

Z

Do not do this exercise if you have a disk problem in your neck. From the Shoulder Stand, bend your knees until they touch your forehead, then slowly straighten your legs over your head until your toes touch the floor (Z). If this is comfortable, you can straighten your arms and place your hands, palms down, on the floor. Hold for several seconds. Relax your breath. To come out of the pose, bend your knees and bring them back to your forehead. Slowly roll forward to a seated position and bend your head forward for a few seconds.

REPETITIONS: 1

Bow Pose

Relieves chronic constipation; improves functioning of digestive system; strengthens back and thigh muscles; increases vitality.

Lie on your stomach with your forehead on the floor and your knees bent. Reach back and grasp your ankles (AA). Breathe out completely, then breathe in and lift up, balancing on your stomach (BB). Look up. Breathe out and lower to the starting position.

REPETITIONS: 3

Turn on your back and rest.

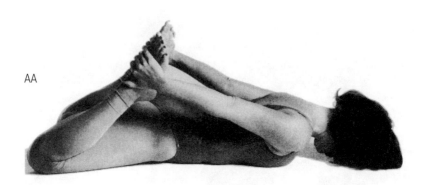

AA

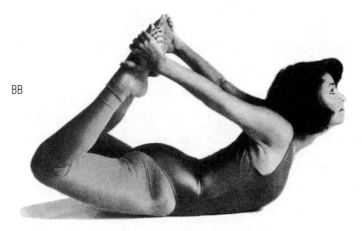

BB

Alternate Toe Touch

Stimulates nerves and muscles in the hips and pelvis; strengthens the legs and lower back.

Lie on your back with legs together and arms overhead on the floor. Breathe out completely, then breathe in and raise your left arm and left leg (CC). Try to touch your toes without lifting your shoulder off the floor. Breathe out and lower the leg and arm. Repeat with the right leg and arm.

REPETITIONS: 3 on each side

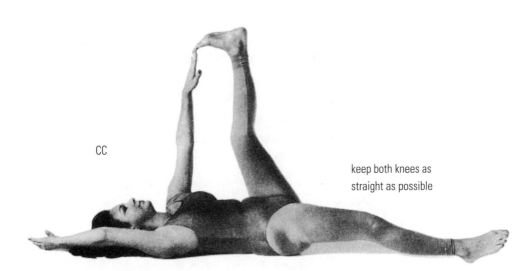

CC

keep both knees as
straight as possible

EASY BRIDGE

Improves functioning of thyroid; eases back pain and fatigue; increases circulation to head.

Lying on your back, bend your knees and bring your feet as close to your hips as possible. Separate your feet several inches. Place your arms, palms down, at your sides. Relax your neck and upper back, breathe out completely, pushing your waist to the floor slightly, then breathe in and raise your hips, arching your back and tucking your chin toward your chest (DD). Hold for 1 or 2

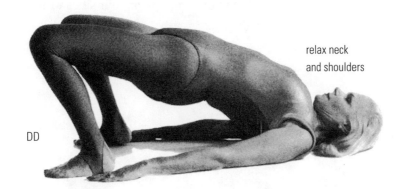

relax neck
and shoulders

DD

seconds, then breathe out and lower. As you become more limber, you can hold on to your ankles for a greater stretch.

REPETITIONS: 3

How to Get the Most Efficient, Relaxed Stretch

When you stretch a muscle nearly to its limit, its automatic reaction is to contract slightly, so that it doesn't tear. This is especially true when you bounce or stretch hard, as in some calisthenic-type exercise routines. In yoga it's important always to stretch slowly and smoothly; most yoga *asana* (poses) also incorporate a particular breathing pattern. Although in a beginning routine you should not hold a pose for more than a few seconds, you can accomplish a lot in those few seconds. When you are stretched to what you think is your limit, consciously relax *into* the stretch, and hold, breathing gently and stopping mental conversation. You'll find that the muscles will release themselves a bit more and you'll get a longer, more relaxed stretch without pain.

BABY POSE
Limbers and relaxes lower back; improves circulation to the brain and pelvic region; improves reproductive and digestive systems' functioning; improves respiration; reduces large stomach.

Sit on your feet with knees together. Slowly bend forward so your head touches the floor. Let your arms rest at your sides with your

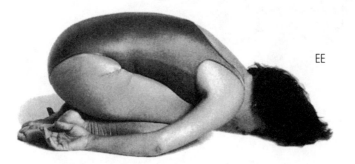

EE

elbows bent so they rest on the floor (EE). This will relax your shoulders and neck. Your head can rest on the forehead or bridge of the nose. Wiggle around a bit to find the most comfortable position. Let your breath relax, and hold for at least a minute. If this position is not comfortable, try resting your head on folded arms; if that is still too uncomfortable, use this position as an exercise, hold it only for a few seconds, then lie down on your back to rest.

REPETITIONS: 1

COBRA POSE

Improves functioning of digestive, respiratory, and reproductive systems; limbers and strengthens entire spine; strengthens eyesight; equalizes two sides of the body; improves complexion.

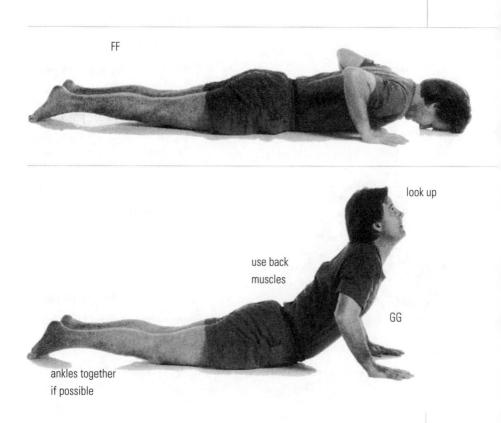

FF

look up

use back
muscles

GG

ankles together
if possible

Lie on your stomach with legs together (those with occasional lower back trouble should separate the legs at first). Place your forehead on the floor and your palms underneath your shoulders, close to your body, so your elbows point up (FF), not out to the sides. Breathe out completely, then start to breathe in as you curl first your head and eyes back as far as they will go, then your chest, and then your stomach. Keep your hipbones on the floor—this is not a push-up—and your arms slightly bent (unless you are extremely limber). Use your back muscles more than your arms. Hold for a few seconds at the top, with your breath in and your eyes looking up through your forehead (GG). Then start to breathe out and curl forward slightly, in reverse; your stomach curls down first, then your chest, and finally your head and eyes. Your eyes are the first part of the body to curl up and the last to curl down.

REPETITIONS: 3

Caution: This is a very powerful exercise and should not be done if you have had recent surgery, if you have an open cut anywhere on your body, or by women during the menstrual period.

TWISTING TRIANGLE

Increases flexibility and circulation in hips and lower back; strengthens hip joints and upper back; helps relieve depression.

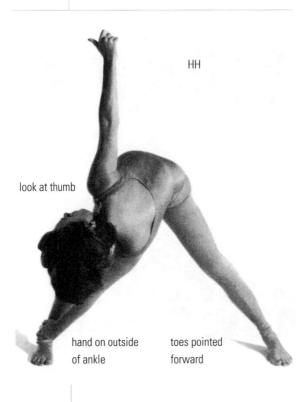

HH

look at thumb

hand on outside
of ankle

toes pointed
forward

Separate your feet as far as you can comfortably (without losing your balance) and point your toes forward. Breathe in, and raise your arms to the sides, parallel to the floor. Breathe out as you bend toward the left leg, grasping the outside of your left ankle (or calf) with your right hand, then turn your head so you are looking at your left hand, which should be pointed straight up, fingers curled and thumb toward you (HH). Stare at your thumb. Pull slightly with your right hand to increase the stretch. Keep both knees straight. Hold for a second or two, then breathe in and come back to your starting position, arms outstretched. Breathe out and repeat to the right leg.

REPETITIONS: 3 on each side
Bring your feet together and stand with eyes closed, body and breathe relaxed, for a few seconds until your breath returns to normal.

TREE POSE

Improves posture, poise, balance, concentration, respiration; strengthens legs.

Stare at one spot on the wall or floor in front of you (but keep your head straight). Breathing normally, slowly raise your right leg and place your right foot as high on the inside of your left leg as possible. Point the toes down and relax the leg; both these suggestions will help keep your

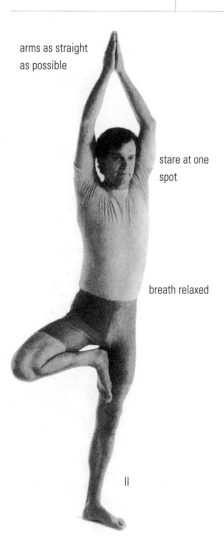

arms as straight as possible

stare at one spot

breath relaxed

II

foot from slipping down your leg. When you feel steady, exhale completely, then slowly breath in and raise your arms over your head. Straighten your arms and place your palms together (II). Now relax your breath and hold the pose for 10 to 30 seconds. Watch for tightness in your stomach muscles, which will tense your breathing. Relax your breath throughout. Keep staring at one spot for balance. Hold for several seconds, then slowly lower arms and leg. Repeat with the other leg. If you have trouble balancing, practice this exercise standing next to a sturdy chair or the wall, and hold on with one hand. It's more important to relax your breath in this balance pose than to raise your arms overhead.

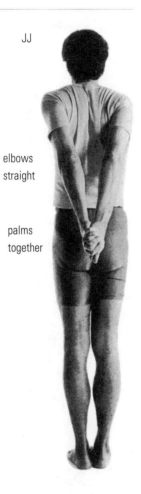

JJ

elbows
straight

palms
together

REPETITIONS: 1 on each side

Full Bend Variation

Improves posture; limbers shoulder joints and upper back vertebrae; improves respiration.

Clasp your hands behind your back and straighten your arms (JJ). If you can, lock your elbows as shown and press your palms together so your shoulder blades are squeezed together as tightly as possible. Breathe in, standing straight, then breathe out and bend forward, keeping your arms pulled back and away from your body (KK). Keep knees straight. Breathe in and straighten back to your starting position. If it is difficult to sustain the arms-locked position for all 3 repetitions, relax your arms, shake them out, and gently roll your head back and forth for a moment between each complete movement.

REPETITIONS: 3

FULL BEND HOLD

Releases tension in the upper back and neck; helps to reduce a large stomach.

After your third Full Bend Variation, breathe out and come forward once again, but let your arms relax toward the floor (LL). If you can reach the floor comfortably, let your fingers curl slightly. Go limp and relax, let your head hang so your neck stretches out a bit, and relax your breath. Hold for several seconds, then slowly stand up. If your lower back is tight, don't hold as long.

REPETITIONS: 1

CAMEL POSE

Limbers entire spine; improves circulation and respiration; stretches

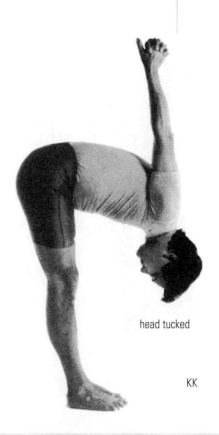

head tucked

KK

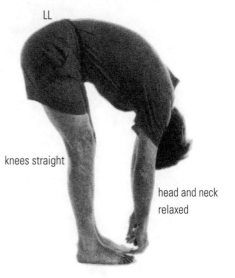

LL

knees straight

head and neck
relaxed

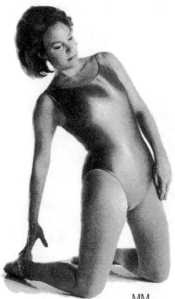

and strengthens thighs and knees; improves functioning of thyroid.

Kneel with legs slightly separated. The first two movements in this exercise help to prepare the spine for an intense stretch. Carefully bend back and grasp your left heel with your left hand. Push your hips forward slightly (MM). Repeat on the right side. Now bend backward and grasp both heels. Push your hips forward as far as possible and let your head relax back (NN). Hold for several seconds, breathing normally. Release and rest briefly in Baby Pose.

MM

REPETITIONS: 1

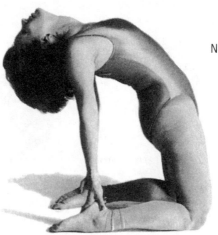

NN

YOGA AT WORK

Here are some stretches that can be done sitting in a straight-back chair. Try these when your energy is lagging at the office. These are much more rejuvenating than a cup of coffee or a snack. Cut out these pages and hang them up near your desk.

SEATED SIDE STRETCH
Limbers spinal column, improves respiration, reduces waistline.

Sitting with your feet slightly apart, breathe in and raise your arms out to the sides. Breathe out and bend toward the left, keeping your arms straight and trying to reach the floor with your left hand (OO). Breathe in, come back to the starting position, then breathe out and bend toward the right.

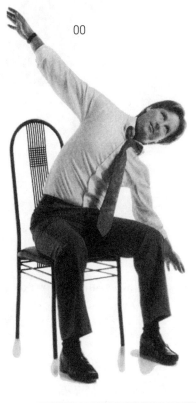

REPETITIONS: 3 on each side

ANKLE ROTATIONS AND POINT-FLEXES
Improves circulation to feet.

Hold on to the seat of your chair, stretch your legs out in front of you, and rotate your ankles several times in each direction. Then point and flex the feet several times.

REPETITIONS: 5–6 circles in each direction, 5–6 point-flexes

SEATED LEG LIFTS
Strengthens legs, hips, and lower back; improves circulation to legs and feet.

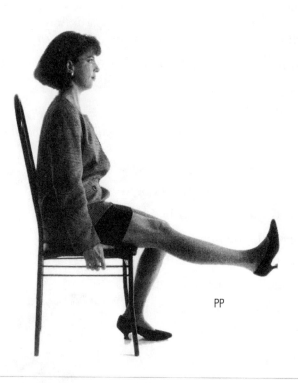

PP

Hold on to the seat of your chair for leverage. Breathe out, then breathe in as you lift your right leg straight, foot flexed (PP). Breathe out and lower your leg.

REPETITIONS: 3 for each leg

Seated Twist

Increases flexibility and circulation in entire spine; improves eyesight.

Sit on the front half of your chair. Place your left hand on the outside of your right knee and hook your right arm over the back of your chair, or inside, as shown. Breathe in, looking forward, then breathe out as you twist to the right. Turn your head and eyes as far right as they will go and stare at a spot just above eye level (QQ). Pull slightly on your right knee with your left hand for more leverage. Relax your breath and hold the position, breathing normally, for several seconds. Release and repeat on the opposite side.

REPETITIONS: 1 on each side

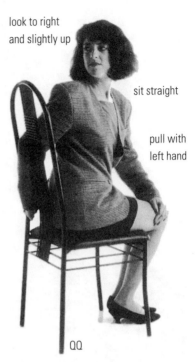

look to right and slightly up

sit straight

pull with left hand

SEATED KNEE SQUEEZE
Limbers and relaxes lower back; improves digestion; improves respiration.

Breathe out completely. Breathe in and lift your right leg with both hands and pull it to your chest while holding your breath in. Tuck your head toward your knee and let your raised foot relax (RR). Hold for a few seconds, then release and switch sides.

REPETITIONS: 3 on each side

QQ

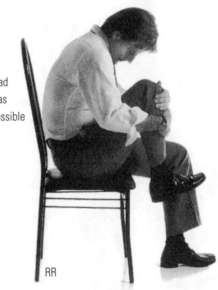

bring head to knee as far as possible

SUN POSE IN CHAIR
Improves circulation to head; massages internal organs; limbers spine and hip joints.

Separate your legs and sit with your hips against the back of the chair. Breathe

RR

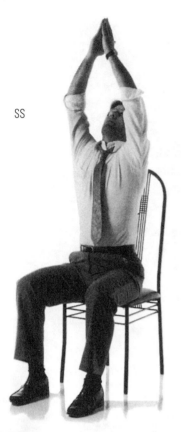

SS

out completely. Breathe in and raise your arms in a circle to the sides and overhead. Look up and stretch (SS). Breathe out, tuck your head, and bend forward between your legs. If you can reach the floor, place your palms flat (TT). Breathe in and raise your arms up over your head again, then breathe out and lower your arms to the sides.

REPETITIONS: 3

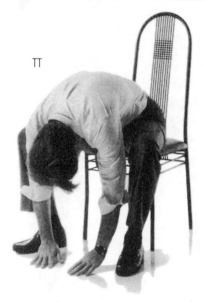

TT

step 3: topical creams, new and old—which ones work to build new skin

The first two steps of my program condition your skin from the inside out. They are vitally important in establishing more youthful skin. Now we move on to the steps that improve your skin from the outside in. Topical solutions are being bioengineered at a breakneck pace, and it is important to understand what is available now, and what is soon to come. This will help you plan your skin care for your lifetime.

Your skin varies in thickness. It is thickest on your palms and the soles of your feet. Your skin is thinnest and most fragile on the face, neck, and hands. You can use soap and water on the rest of your body (I like nonsoap pH-balanced cleansers such as Oil of Olay and Neutrogena), but your thin skin needs more gentle treatment. The face and neck should be maintained with extra-protective topical moisturizing creams. This is where the array of products can be overwhelming. Some of the active ingredients are enormously effective, but some are too diluted in strength to have much effect at all. Still others are simply ineffectual gimmicks, so that their makers can charge you more money for a "miracle cream" that is nothing stronger than baby lotion.

The information in this chapter applies to patients with all skin types: Caucasian, African-American, Asian, and Latino complexions. In my experience, melanin content may determine the color of your skin, but the key difference in skin types is your genetic history, and whether your skin is oily, normal, or dry.

Cleansing for Normal to Dry Skin

You should wash your face in the morning and in the evening. If your skin is very dry, you may wish to cleanse it only in the evening and skip the morning. Rinse your face many times, particularly if you wear makeup. Soap can be drying, so a nonsoap cleansing cream is best for most skin types. The skin's normal pH balance is on the acidic side, and soap tends to be more alkaline. Getting that "squeaky clean" feeling is actually not good for your skin—over time, it can even make your skin thinner. Good cleanser brands are Cetaphil, Basis, Purpose, Neutrogena, Oil of Olay, and fragrance-free Dove. These are easily found in drugstores and supermarkets. If you prefer more expensive, department-store brands, stick with Clé de Peau and Kanebo cleansers suited to your skin type.

The Proper pH

pH stands for potential hydrogen, and refers to the amount of acid or alkaline in a liquid. This measurement is used by horticulturists to maintain healthy soil for plants. It also applies to the treatment of your skin to maintain glowing health. The pH scale is 0 to 14—anything below the midpoint of 7 is considered an acid. Anything over 7 is alkaline. Normal skin has a pH between 4 and 6, ideally at 5.5. That means your skin is more on the acid side. Your skin uses this acid, combined in a delicate balance with your perspiration, to retain moisture while not allowing bacteria into your pores.

Most soaps have a pH higher than 8, but certain cleansers are more balanced. Cleansers recommended by dermatologists have a low pH. Good brands that are easily available include Cetaphil and Purpose.

Cleansing for Oily or Acne-Prone Skin

Many adults still suffer from enlarged pores and oily skin, particularly those with a Mediterranean or Latino complexion. Other adults suffer from acne. Comedones, or blocked pores, are often the basis of acne. You should continue using the acne control medication that works for you, when you get breakouts. Good brands are Clearasil and Neutrogena, or those prescribed by a dermatologist.

Some cleansers, moisturizers, and makeup products cause comedones because they contain ingredients such as oils, wax, fatty acids, or esters. These elements help "spread" the product on your skin. When you see the term "noncomedogenic," it means the product does not contain these harmful agents. However, some patients have skin that responds well to such oils, if used sparingly. Some people, using certain comedogenic products, find they dissolve facial oil because they are similar elements. Whenever you purchase cleansers, toners, moisturizers, night creams, foundation, blush, or sunscreens, be aware of these elements:

Highly Comedogenic Ingredients

Linseed oil	Olive oil	Cocoa butter	Oleic acid
Coal tar	Isopropyl	Squalene	Oleyl alcohol
Isopropyl	isostearate	Acetylated	Lanolic acid
myristate	Mysteryl	lanolin	Butyl stearate
Isopropyl	myristate	Myreth 3	
palmitate	Isopropyl	myristate	
	linoleate		

Moderately Comedogenic Ingredients
(usually not a problem when used in diluted forms)

Decyl oleate	Sorbitan oleate	Myristyl lactate
Coconut oil	Grape seed oil	Sesame oil
Hexylene glycol	Isostearyl neopentanoate	Tocopherol
Most D and C red dyes	Octyldodecanol	Peanut oil
Lauric acid	Mink oil	Corn oil
Safflower oil	Lauryl alcohol	Lanolin alcohol
Glycerin stearate	Lanolin	Sunflower oil
Avocado oil	Mineral oil	

Noncomedogenic Ingredients

Glycerin	Squalane	Sorbitol
Sodium PCA	Zinc stearate	SD alcohol
Allantoin	Propylene	Octyldodecyl stearate
Butylene glycol	glycol	Panthenol
Dimethicone	Polysorbates	Water
Iron oxides	Jojoba oil	Petrolatum

Cyclomethicone	Cetyl palmate	Octylmethoxycinnimate
Oxybenzone	Isopropyl alcohol	Sodium hyaluronate
Tridecyl trimellitate	Phenyl trimethicone	Tridecyl stearate
Propylene glycol dicaprate/ dicaprylate	Octyldodecyl stearoyl stearate	

Mild exfoliation is good for your complexion. It stimulates blood circulation to your face, and sloughs off dead skin cells, leaving a smooth, refreshed surface. Don't use loofahs or rough buffers on your face, however. Between their harshness and their bacterial content, these can cause more problems than they do improvement. Bacteria cause acne, as well as rosacea. The best way to exfoliate while you are cleansing is to use a clean cotton cloth—a washcloth. Gently apply skin cleanser to the cloth, and rub gently on your face, neck, and upper chest. Do not use the cloth a second time without washing it. Either launder it thoroughly with bleach, or invest in disposable cleansing cloths.

Mild masks and granular scrubs are acceptable, but be cautious with them. I like the gentle ones you can usually find at a salon or spa. As with facial waxing, masks are not recommended for those using Accutane or Retin-A, or if you have rosacea or acne, as they are irritating. Patients who have dark skin are also more susceptible to irritation from scrubbing.

If you have tight, dry skin, or oily, acne-prone skin, a salon might also offer a facial mask called an "enzyme treatment" to exfoliate your complexion. These are usually quite gentle. A salon might also offer alpha hydroxy or glycolic acid peels, which are low-strength peeling procedures. These "superficial peels" are usually very beneficial if your skin is not overly sensitive. They basically serve as a chemical exfoliant. There are stronger peels that do more than exfoliate, and all of the peels are described in Chapter 5.

This skin condition strikes more than 13 million Americans, and appears as redness in the cheeks, nose, chin, and forehead. It is often genetic, and usually strikes an adult after the age of thirty. If rosacea is left untreated, the redness can become permanent, and more dilated blood vessels may appear. Doctors frequently prescribe antibiotics to help clear outbreaks, but there are a number of prescription cleansers and creams to control this condition without medication. Some of the more effective products are Metrogel, Nizoral, and Plurion. Special cleansers are available over the counter that can help relieve rosacea, such as Cetaphil, Oilatum AD, and fragrance-free Dove.

Do not let this condition go untreated. It can be worsened by stress, sun exposure, alcohol consumption, spicy food, exercise, certain prescription drugs, overly zealous facial cleansing, and the use of Retin-A. If you have a friend who has signs of redness, or who blushes excessively, ask her to consult a doctor.

How to Wash Your Face

- Put a dime-sized amount of mild cleanser in the palm of your hand.
- Rub on your face for fifteen seconds or so, using your fingertips or gently with a cloth.
- Rinse your face again and again—ten times—using water that is just tepid.
- Rinse a couple times more.
- Pat with a clean towel.

Tone

When I talk about "toning" skin, I am referring to the use of an astringent that prepares the skin for treatment. Toners rid excess cleanser and oils from your face and gently dilate blood vessels. One of my favorite products is plain old witch hazel, which costs about two dollars a bottle in any drugstore. Other toners contain alcohol, which can cause excessive dryness. If you can find a brand that does not contain alcohol, you might give it a try. But none is superior to the effects of witch hazel.

Treat

Before you apply sunscreen, you should choose a topical treatment to retain or replenish moisture and volume to your complexion. As with body lotions, many moisturizers are very similar in effectiveness. Good, basic moisturizers include Avon, Nivea Visage, Neutrogena Healthy Skin, L'Oréal Plenitude, and Oil of Olay ProVital.

Be aware that some moisturizers are comedogenic, particularly if you have oily skin. There are wonderful oil-free moisturizers from Complex 15, Purpose, and Neutrogena Healthy Skin. And many moisturizers are now enhanced with antiaging molecules for extra treatment.

Retin-A, also called *tretinoin* or *retinoic acid,* is the vitamin A acid that was developed in the 1960s by Dr. Albert Kligman at the University of Pennsylvania. This cream helps unblock the follicles, stimulates collagen production, and is a drying agent used for acne and oily skin. While alpha hydroxy acids work on the surface of your skin, tretinoin directly affects a cell's nucleus, regulating genetic activity to recharge cell division and production of new collagen. Over the years, it has proved to firm up skin and reduce wrinkles, roughness, and freckles. It is a powerful *keratolytic,* which means it increases the skin's collagen-makers, keratinocytes and fibroblasts. Tretinoin dissolves proteins—the dirt and debris in your pores—so it can be irritating to some patients. Most new clients experience redness and flaking, so it is used sparingly to start. Because it makes your skin more vulnerable to the sun's damaging rays, most people should use it at bedtime. Some prefer the products known as Avita, Differin, Retin-A Micro, or Renova because they contain more moisturizers than Retin-A. Certain over-the-counter products contain something called Retinol, a weakened derivative of Vitamin A. Retinol has less effectiveness than Retin-A or Renova. While Retinol products are fine for your skin, you simply won't see the same results.

As effective as it can be, Retin-A is not for everyone. Some believe that it decreases wrinkles by causing a low-grade inflammation of the dermis with chronic swelling. This constant swelling may reduce wrinkles, but it is not healthy to maintain chronic inflammation of any kind. Chronic inflammation can actually accelerate the aging process. Unless there is a medical indication for long-term use of Retin-A, such as acne or keratoses, I do not advise patients to use Retin-A or Renova for more than a few months at a time. In other words, take a Retin-A "holiday." Patients with rosacea should not use Retin-A at all, as it can dilate the blood vessels and make redness worse.

If you are using Retin-A for purely aesthetic reasons, be sure to rotate off this medication for part of the year. Also, it is recommended that other keratolytic agents, such as benzoyl peroxide, salicylic acid, and glycolic acid, be removed from your regimen if you are using Retin-A. I would also not recommend using products that contain alcohol, such as astringents, exfoliants, and masks. Facial waxing is also not recommended for Retin-A patients. Use electrolysis or lasers to continue your hair removal regimen. Retin-A can show results in just three months, if used on a daily basis. Use of sunscreen is imperative when using Retin-A, and I often recommend that women simply not use this cream in the summer months.

Another derivative of vitamin A is Accutane, a potent oral supplement used to control acne. Accutane must be used only with a doctor's close supervision. It is a very effective product, although it is known to cause birth defects, so it is not prescribed to women who are or might become pregnant. Users of this product must take even more care to avoid the sun, increasing the use of sunscreens. And patients using this drug may not have any aesthetic surgical or peeling procedure on their faces until they cease taking it for an entire year. In fact, prior to getting *any* procedure, such as a laser, chemical peel, or dermabrasion, patients should stop using Accutane for at least one year.

Adapalene is a compound with similar properties as retinoic acid, but it is much milder and often less irritating to patients. Another alternative to Retin-A is the adapalene cream known as Differin.

Alpha hydroxy acid (or *AHA,* derived from citrus fruits), *beta hydroxy acid* (also known as *salicylic acid,* derived from willow bark), and *lactic acid* (from milk) can improve the hydration and firmness of your skin, as well as even out your skin's color. Look for a product that has 8 to 10 percent acid, and a pH of 3.5 or less. These acids do not reverse sun damage, but they have a nice effect on improving your skin cells. I find that some patients tolerate one of these acids better than the others. Julie G., for example, found that products containing salicylic acid made her break out with acne from blocked pores. AHAs had no such effect on her complexion.

When they appeared in the 1980s, AHA creams were an early step into twenty-first-century skin care. They were the first effective ingredients added to skin creams that actually did something other than merely moisturize. Back in Cleopatra's day, she knew the power of this acid when she took milk baths to soften her skin. All AHAs are keratolytic and act as a biochemical buffer.

For all-over body care, I recommend AHA creams, which are available in many affordable lotions from numerous manufacturers. These AHA acids are essentially exfoliants, which speed up the process of sloughing off dead skin cells. One study from 1993 revealed that using an AHA cream in conjunction with a retinoic acid increased the benefits of both elements—the two creams together were more powerful than "the sum of their parts." This proved particularly noticeable in patients who were in their fifties or older. It seems the properties of AHAs increase the body's tolerance for stronger doses of tretinoin.

Azelaic acid, in a prescription cream called Azelex, is a substance derived from grain, a natural exfoliant that also corrects pigment spots and relieves acne. It is more potent than glycolic acid, and works as well as hydroquinone to reduce age spots. If your skin does not respond well to Retin-A or hydroquinone, ask your doctor to prescribe Azelex.

Vitamin C (also known as ascorbic acid) is often used as a topical antioxidant in a clear serum form. Some researchers believe antioxidants reduce enzymes that damage collagen and repel free radicals. Free radicals are unstable oxygen molecules that have an extra electron. They are naturally produced by the body's chemical interactions, and excessively produced by sun exposure, poor diet, and smoking. Because they are unstable, free radicals unload the extra electron by binding it to our skin's collagen, elastin, and DNA, which are then damaged by this extra electron. Over time, the millions of these free radicals wreak havoc with your skin. Antioxidants act like a vacuum cleaner with free radicals, sweeping them up and inactivating them. Topical brands, which do not require a prescription, include Cellex-C and Citrix. It has a very short shelf life—it loses its effectiveness within eight weeks of opening the jar. And it also loses its effectiveness quickly after it's applied to your skin—even as quickly as twenty minutes. I have developed a form of vitamin C that is made without any water (anhydrous), has a significantly increased shelf life, and is effective on the skin for up to twelve hours. Our special form of long-acting vitamin C is contained in RéVive's Arrête Booster C.

In addition to vitamin C, another great antioxidant is *superoxide dismutase* (SOD). This is what makes white blood cells so powerful in fighting off disease. In many instances SOD is more potent and more stable than vitamin C. SOD is contained in my RéVive night cream known as Serum Prôtectif.

Vitamin E, or *tocopherol,* is also considered an antioxidant, and topical use prevents the formation of dark age spots. When taken orally, vitamin E decreases the "stickiness" of platelets, which can be great for people with cardiovascular disease. It must always be stopped three weeks before any surgery, however, as it can cause excessive bleeding.

Hydroquinone cream contains a melanin suppressant that reverses the dark patches of skin caused by aging. There are several types of bleaching agents, but hydroquinone is probably the most commonly known. Sun spots, also known as melasma, lentigines, or hyperpigmentation, start to occur in your complexion when you're in your twenties. (Freckles are formed in childhood.) Hydroquinone is a plant-derived product that, in effect, "bleaches" the skin back to a more uniform color. Over-the-counter brands are half as strong as the prescription creams. It takes several months before you notice any fading, and, as with other potent creams, I do not believe it should be used for more than four to six months at a stretch. Your skin needs a break from time to time.

I prefer the prescription brands Lustra-AF and Tri-Luma. Hydroquinone creams are more effective when they are used in tandem with Retin-A because, together, they inhibit the production of melanin.

There is a prescription treatment known as Obagi cream that combines hydroquinone with tretinoin and alpha hydroxy acids. This powerful combination has a positive effect on smoothing out your skin and eliminating pigment spots. Once it is stopped, however, the skin reverts to its previous pattern. Many of these creams do not have lasting effects, and only show improvement while you are using them. Obagi is intense and, like Retin-A, it is not for everyone and should *never* be used for more than a nine-to-twelve-month period.

Kinerase is a plant-derived prescription cream that contains kinetin. It is a plant growth factor that stimulates cell division in plants and prevents the aging of leaves. In humans, it is said to stimulate fibroblasts, the cells that produce collagen. There are commercial skin lotions that contain collagen, but collagen molecules are too large to penetrate the skin. Kinerase supposedly penetrates the skin and allegedly prompts skin cells to make more collagen. However, it is a plant growth factor. In my opinion, it just can't have the effects of a human growth factor. Plant molecules don't work on human cells. They work on plant cells.

I mentioned commercial products that contain *retinol*, the highly diminuted form of Retin-A. Products containing retinol are primarily moisturizers, but may have slightly more potency than regular moisturizers. The same is true for creams containing the coenzyme Q_{10} and *copper*, or natural elements such as *alpha lipoic acid* or *DMAE*. The creams are good moisturizing products that contain trace amounts of antioxidants to repel free radicals, but they are not the magic creams promoters claim them to be.

The Japanese use other compounds to keep their skin fresh and even-toned. One of them is *arbutin,* a product derived from the leaves of pear trees. Rather than bleaching the skin, arbutin seems to prevent future spots from forming. *Kojic acid* is derived from a fungus called aspergillis, and is used as a food additive to keep food fresh. Kojic acid is a popular skin whitener in Japan, and it is available in a number of American products, although it is expensive. Some patients are allergic to kojic acid, but it has a long shelf life. Almost any skin whitener or "bleach" implements change by blocking the conversion of your body's amino acids (specifically, the one known as tyrosine) into melanin. Often, this compound is combined in a cosmetic with a skin brightener that, in effect, reflects sunlight to make your face seem lighter.

A plant-based peptide called Pal-KTTKS has been marketed in a cream called StriVectin SD. It has been shown in clinical studies to reduce the depth, length, roughness, and discoloration of stretch marks. Consumers started putting this cream on their faces, and found that it reduced fine lines and wrinkles. After the manufacturer went back to the lab to test its effects on the face, they learned that the skin was slightly thickened. StriVectin performed better than retinol, vitamin C, and a placebo. This same botanical peptide is contained in a cream called TYK Energy Renewal Revelation. Again, I am very skeptical of plant molecules affecting skin, except for moisturization or irritation. There simply are *not* receptors on human cell surfaces for plant molecules. Our bodies' immune systems recognize plant molecules as foreign. Small amounts of irritation can result in a perceived improvement in skin because of low-grade swelling; however, over time this can prove to be deleterious. Think of poison ivy as the extreme. Human skin cells do *not* have receptors for plant molecules; human skin cells have receptors for human molecules.

The sun's ultraviolet rays are classified into UVC (the least harmful, largely blocked by the ozone layer), UVB (which cause sunburns and some skin cancers), and UVA (longer waves that are more insidious because they do not cause burning but do cause DNA mutation, which can lead to cancer. UVA rays are commonly used in tanning bed machines). All of these rays cause DNA damage. In only a couple of decades, skin shows the effects of UV rays, even if you never go to the beach.

The dangers of skin cancer from sun exposure exist for a lifetime, and they are cumulative, even if you curtailed sunbathing when you were younger. Some experts claim that 80 percent of the sun's lifetime damage occurs in our first eighteen years of life, most of it not from sunbathing but from day-to-day exposure. I think it's closer to 40 percent, because you spend further decades in the sun, simply while running errands or working in the yard. Even on a short-term basis, the sun essentially bakes your skin, drying it out like crackers in an oven. The sun can cause hyperpigmentation—age spots—in someone as young as twenty-two. Adding to the negative effects of sun exposure is the damage caused by free radical molecules. These chemical pollutants injure skin cells and accumulate over time to cause wrinkles, age spots, and rough skin.

There are three basic types of skin cancer: *Basal cell carcinoma* is the most common, and is frequently located in parts of the body with greater sun exposure—the face, hands, legs, arms, and back. These only grow locally and do not spread (metastasize) to other sites. These are small, pearl-like growths under the skin that are very curable with treatment from a dermatologist. *Squamous cell carcinoma* is similar to basal cell but it can spread farther and more quickly. It appears as a red bump on your skin, like a wound that won't heal. *Melanoma* is the most dangerous. It appears as a dark mole—commonly identified by the Skin Cancer Institute's "ABCD's of Melanoma." This acronym is short for "Asymmetric," or uneven, one-sided growth; a "Border" that is bumpy or unclear; "Color" that is dark brown or blotchy multicolored; and a "Diameter" the size of a pencil eraser or larger. Regular moles are smaller. An annual visit to a dermatologist will keep you safe from serious skin cancer.

Tanning booths cause the same skin cancers and damage as regular exposure to the sun. Some over-the-counter pills claim to promote self-tanning by using a chemical called canthaxanthin. As the side effects of this drug are not known, I do not recommend it. For those who enjoy having a suntan, there are a number of new self-tanning products and application procedures available in salons that produce spectacular results—the "buff 'n' bronze" or the all-over misting shower. They are harmless to your skin, and they last several days. I don't see the point in choosing anything but self-tanners if you care about looking good in the long term.

If you do nothing else for your skin, use a sunscreen. These creams contain safe chemicals that neutralize ultraviolet light, and are now frequently found in daily moisturizers and foundation makeup. Today's commercial products are very effective but the average person never uses enough. Unlike moisturizers, the brands of sunscreens vary widely in effectiveness. You need a "broad spectrum" product to block all three of the sun's harmful rays. The most effective chemical that provides broad spectrum protection is called avobenzone (also called Parsol 1789), and it is found in many sunscreen products. The higher the Sun Protection Factor (SPF) rating, the more effective the sunblock. The SPF of 15 blocks about 94 percent of UVB rays, whereas an SPF 30 blocks about 98 percent. Waterproof sunscreens contain extra oils or fats to make them resistant to water. They will block your pores, but this is usually acceptable if you don't use them on your face. If you have extremely sensitive skin, you may want to use the old-fashioned zinc-oxide creams, or titanium dioxide. They are no longer brilliant white, but come in a variety of transparent shades. Most drugstores, for example, sell a very inexpensive jar of hypoallergenic clear zinc oxide that has a 45 SPF. Solbar makes transparent zinc in a tube that has an SPF of 38. It's waterproof and noncomedogenic. It still needs to be applied thirty minutes before going out into the sun.

Many people disregard these directions on the back of the bottle: Always apply sunscreen *thirty minutes before* going out into the sun. It actually takes the cream this long to penetrate the epidermis and become activated.

Many of us inherit our sun sensitivity from our parents—and many of us are affected by living closer to the equator than other people. Regardless of where you live, you should use sunscreen on the exposed parts of your body all year long, rain or shine. African Americans, Asians, and Latinos are also susceptible to sun damage. The added melanin (pigment) in these skin types protects you more than fair-skinned people, but not completely. Even if you wear light clothing or a sun hat, you should apply liberal amounts of sunscreen. The sun can penetrate fabric and reflect off of a hat brim. Walk in the shade whenever you can, and stay away from direct sunlight, even indoors, and especially between 11:00 A.M. and 3:00 P.M. Applying extra moisturizers after sun exposure does not counteract the sun's damage. Only a sunscreen, applied *before* sun exposure, can do that.

Since your body benefits from all-over moisturizing creams, save a step and buy ones that already have sunscreen. Although the creams that contain alpha hydroxy acid are great for your skin, you then have to add a layer of sunscreen over them. Good brands that combine sunscreen with moisturizers include Lubriderm Daily UV Lotion and Eucerin Daily Sun Defense. Alternatively, you can simply use a good sunscreen as a body lotion. Sunscreens from Shade, Neutrogena, Coppertone, Banana Boat, and No-Ad typically range up to SPF 45. They offer great conditioners for all-over skin care. You may use them on your face, but be aware that most of them are comedogenic.

Moisturizing your skin is essential, even if the lotion does not contain sunscreen. I like brands such as Aveeno, Avon, Eucerin, Keri, Lubriderm, and Nivea. You need not choose the expensive brands at department stores to get a smoothing effect all over your body. Taking care of your whole body, inside and out, shows in your face. Your face sees more sun than any other part of your body, and people see your face more than they do the rest of you. Therefore, your face needs special attention.

One of the most important beauty treatments you should perform regularly is this: Apply sunscreen to your face, neck, and hands—once in the morning, and then again at lunchtime. Many makeup foundations and blushes contain sunscreen now, but don't be fooled into thinking that's enough protection. Most skin cancers grow on the perimeter of the face, which you may inadvertently miss! As with body skin care, I have found some superb facial moisturizers that already contain sunscreen, saving you a step in your skin care regimen. These include:

- Eucerin Extra Protective Moisturizing Lotion—SPF 30

- Neutrogena Healthy Defense Daily Moisturizer—SPF 30

- RoC Age-Diminishing Daily Moisturizer—SPF 15

- Aveeno Skin Positively Radiant Daily Moisturizer, or Brightening Daily Treatment—SPF 15

- Purpose Dual Treatment Lotion, or Intensive Daily Moisturizer—SPF 15

- L'Oréal Dermo-Expertise Line Eraser—SPF 15

- Olay Complete Total Effects, or Age Defying Protective Renewal Lotion—SPF 15

Naturally, you may choose to use any number of other non-sunscreen facial moisturizers at night. You don't need sunscreen at bedtime! The list of great products is extensive. I like products from Clinique, Neutrogena, Oil of Olay, Prescriptives, and Shiseido. These manufacturers specialize in mild yet effective moisturizers.

Step 3, in a Nutshell

- Cleanse and tone your skin repeatedly through the day.
- Choose an advanced topical treatment that works best for your skin. If you have oily or acne-prone skin, try a gel formula. If your skin is sensitive or dry, Renova or Retin-A Micro contains moisturizers. Add to this a bleaching agent, such as hydroquinone cream. Galderma manufactures a prescription cream called Tri-Luma, which contains both tretinoin and hydroquinone, as well as fluocinolone acetonide, which prevents irritation. Your doctor will help you determine which cream works best for you.
- Apply sunscreen in the morning and again at lunchtime. Look for inexpensive brands, or stick to the new clear zinc oxides.

In my clinical studies over the years, I have analyzed—and personally used—most of the facial products available in the United States. Along the way, I discovered a new active ingredient, one that would change the normal life cycle of the human skin cell and actually decrease the aging process of skin.

The Advent of Bioengineering That Builds New Skin at the Cellular Level

Epidermal Growth Factor (EGF) is a natural protein hormone produced by the human body to heal skin injuries. Growth factors exist in all animals and plant life. Some of the plant growth factors have been used in cosmetic creams such as Kinerase, Ahava, and Natura Bissé. These are nice organic moisturizers but, as I mentioned earlier, growth factors in plants and animals are very different from those in humans. They have virtually no effect on human skin. Plant and animal hormones simply cannot interact with human skin cells, despite the claims of marketing companies. Their basic genetic composition prevents them from attaching to human-cell surface receptors.

EGF is a human protein, one of thirty-two known human growth factors. At the time EGF was first isolated in the 1960s, researchers also discovered that human cells on the skin's surface contain the *receptors* for EGF. This means the biological "message" is not only sent but properly received by the cells, telling them to begin action, to divide and replicate themselves. When a person is cut or burned, EGF is naturally released, and skin cells in the affected area start producing identical, healthy cells to replace the injured ones. EGF doesn't change the skin cell, it merely enhances the production of new cells. Making new cells is what healthy skin is all about. The youthful complexion is merely the reflection of vibrant young skin cells being actively replenished.

Doctors have known about EGF for a long time, but we could never obtain enough of the protein to perform clinical tests. The natural concentrations in the body are minuscule—EGF is measured in nanograms, or billionths of a single gram. Modern medical research was young in the 1960s, and technology was still rather crude. That was when Dr. Stanley Cohen extracted EGF from the salivary glands of mice, where it is found in the highest concentrations. All animals, including humans, have EGF in their salivary glands, which may help explain why dogs and cats heal faster when they lick their wounds. In those early years, great quantities of human EGF were very difficult to obtain. Dr. Cohen eventually won the Nobel Prize for discovering EGF, but it wasn't until the 1980s that the bioengineered manufacture of this protein allowed for much greater quantities to be produced for practical applications. After scientists were able to manufacture EGF using recombinant DNA technologies, we finally were able to test EGF and witness its amazing effects.

I was in the right place at the right time. In the early 1980s, I completed my surgical residency and formed a business partnership with a small biotechnical start-up company called Chiron, Inc. Chiron was originally a garage operation in the Bay Area, with four molecular biologists from the University of California. We were all looking at technological advances that could enhance the healing process of skin. After so many years of performing surgery and scar treatments, I had become very familiar with how the skin reacted to every product and procedure.

The scientists at Chiron first manufactured Epidermal Growth Factor by placing its human genome into yeast cells. These yeast cells then started behaving like tiny EGF factories, churning out large quantities of the human protein. Recombinant DNA can only be reproduced by another organism, and yeast fits the bill. Working with the bioengineered EGF, I began ten years of clinical testing. At last, Chiron provided virtually unlimited quantities of EGF for me to use. The clinical trials on human subjects took place in hospitals at Emory and Vanderbilt Universities.

Cure for Wounded Skin

It was very gratifying to see the effects of EGF on damaged skin for the first time. I'll never forget one of my patients, Chloe M., a twenty-five-year-old woman who had been badly burned in a car accident. Her second- and third-degree burns covered about one-third of her body. She was scheduled for a lengthy, painful program of skin graft procedures. After her first surgery, I asked if she would be willing to be a test subject for the new protein from Chiron, and she agreed. I have learned that burn victims will usually try *anything* that promises to alleviate their pain and help them to heal. EGF performed exceptionally. Chloe's burned skin began to regenerate without any further skin grafts at all—a miracle! Even better, the scars were minimal and her skin functioned as well as her original, undamaged skin.

Another patient of mine, James H., was a forty-five-year-old mason whose foot had been amputated due to diabetes. The stump was not healing well and, after six months, it looked as though he was going to have to have another amputation above the knee, to stave off a major infection. I was able to treat his stump with EGF, and it healed within three weeks. His scar was clean and he returned to good health (he still had diabetes, but his other leg was saved, and he was able to walk without pain with his new prosthesis). EGF achieved a seemingly unbelievable cure for James that his doctors had, initially, all but ruled out.

The results of my EGF studies were published in the *New England Journal of Medicine* in 1989. In the meantime, I continued doing my own tests with EGF. Instead of using it in blind tests on patients with burns and wounds, I started using EGF with patients who had no injuries at all. The only thing "wrong" with these test subjects was that their skin was aging normally. These were patients who initially came to me for an aesthetic surgical procedure. When I told them about EGF, they agreed to test the product before resorting to surgery. This was an informal study with volunteers, done in tandem with my clinical healing tests. However, my own studies confirmed for me an equally impressive effect of EGF on normal aging skin.

Cure for Aging Skin

Over the years, it had become evident that the healing of a wound and the reversal of aging skin involve a very similar process in many ways. Both require increased rates of cellular division for a positive outcome. Through cellular division, the epidermis regenerates itself outward from its deepest layer. The new cells rise to the surface and they are imperceptibly sloughed off every day, millions of cells at a time. When a woman is twenty years old, this process requires about three weeks. When she is fifty years old, it takes closer to three months. What we see in older people are, essentially, skin cells that are three months old—or older—instead of the three-week-old complexion of youth. Doctors refer to this middle-aged complexion as *senescent* (from the Latin for "aging") skin.

We had already recognized other aspects of physical aging, such as basal metabolic rate (BMR), which is the speed at which your body burns energy. It takes fewer calories at age forty to keep us alive and healthy than it did when we were twenty. That is why we cannot eat the same way in middle age as we did in our twenties, or we will certainly gain weight. I wondered if the same weren't also true for skin. It, too, behaves differently as we age. I suspected that stimulating cell division in senescent skin would reverse many of the physical signs of aging.

Plastic surgery provided ample opportunities for my detailed research on EGF as a topical cream. Many patients were interested in testing it, as an alternative to aesthetic surgery, and EGF had no known side effects. We were simply enhancing the body's natural regenerative system. To my knowledge, no other aesthetic surgeon was doing any such studies with EGF.

After a few years of using it in my practice, I was able to see that EGF worked as well as I'd surmised. I now see that EGF application has the potential to replace surgery as the optimal treatment for aging skin, in many instances. In addition to its effectiveness on the face, EGF can be used on the neck and hands, and other parts of the body that are not amenable to plastic surgery. I observed that EGF consistently stimulates sluggish cells of aging skin to regenerate more quickly, making skin not only appear younger but physiologically act younger. It *is* younger. At any given time, the EGF-treated skin cell is closer to its infantile stage of division, because it is being replaced more quickly.

We put EGF in a cream, and tested it on hundreds of patients. Reeves L. was a fifty-five-year-old woman who came in to consult with me about a face-lift. She was a successful executive who had always taken good care of her skin, but she was becoming bothered by her crow's-feet and age spots. I asked Reeves if she would like to test a topical protein before planning the surgery. She agreed, and I gave her EGF in a cream that was the prototype for RéVive. After four weeks, her skin was glowing. Her wrinkles had not completely disappeared, but the skin under her eyes was filled with healthy fluid and her complexion was much smoother. Now, at age sixty, Reeves looks better than she did at forty-five. And she no longer feels the need for a face-lift.

When Melanie J. told me she was forty years old, I was surprised. This wife and mother looked much older, with sagging skin and puffy eyes. She was investigating a face-peel to invigorate her appearance, and I suggested the EGF study instead. In ten weeks, Melanie's face looked like she was only twenty-five. Her skin tone was even, and nearly flawless. She said both she and her husband couldn't believe the change in her appearance.

Wendy A. came to see me because she had had a surgical procedure elsewhere eight months earlier that had left two small scars on her forehead. She was not happy with the results of the surgery, and was despairing about the scars. Rather than perform another surgery to repair the damage, I applied EGF to the scars, and to other parts of Wendy's face. Her skin began to regain a healthy glow, and we were able to repair the damaged skin without any further procedures.

Marina S. was a seventy-five-year-old woman who simply wanted to look younger. She was in good health and felt her sagging face didn't reflect her true vitality. Older women experience the greatest degrees of skin change after using EGF. Marina's face became brighter and reacquired a healthy glow she hadn't seen in years.

With the evidence provided by cases like these over the years, I patented cosmetic EGF as an antiaging cream, and launched a product called RéVive in 1997. RéVive is the only cosmetic in the world that contains human EGF, so my references to EGF naturally refer to RéVive. Because EGF does not alter the structure of skin cells, it is not considered a drug that needs to be federally regulated. EGF in RéVive simply enhances the production of new cells.

The results of my EGF treatments speak for themselves. Here are some before-and-after photos of patients who used RéVive for six weeks.

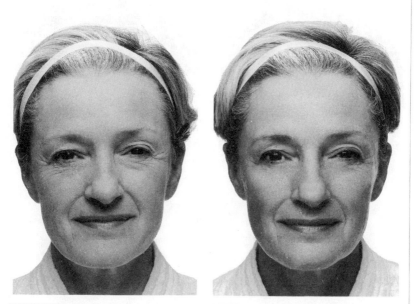

BEFORE RéVive application   AFTER 6 weeks of RéVive application

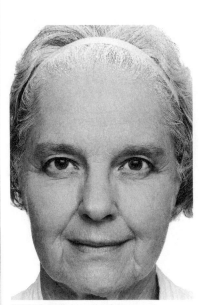

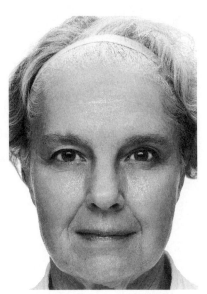

BEFORE RéVive application

AFTER 6 weeks of RéVive application

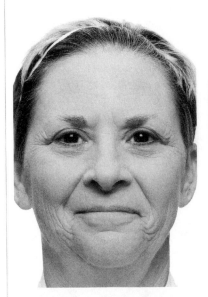

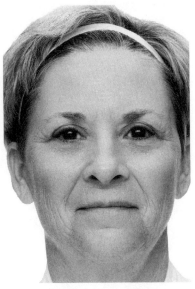

BEFORE RéVive application

AFTER 6 weeks of RéVive application

Some might question the long-term effects of increased skin cell division. I personally supervise patients who have used EGF for up to twenty years, including myself and my mother. None has experienced ill effects. And all of them look younger than they really are.

Does this skin care product also heal burns and wounded skin? Absolutely. We have seen RéVive speed the healing of rosacea, cuts, acne, and any scar on the body that is less than two years old. Two years is the time span in which scars undergo the greatest change. EGF brings new skin to the surface that is literally younger than ever. This change is most noticeable in patients who show the most signs of aging, that is, those who may be older and have more wrinkles. Less damaged or younger women still have young-acting skin. Aged skin doesn't necessarily lose all its wrinkles, but their appearance is noticeably softened, and the overall quality of the skin is remarkably improved. The skin is, indeed, physiologically younger than it was before.

Dozens of cosmetics companies market ineffective products using the same adjectives for younger-looking skin, but none of their claims are based on bioengineered ingredients and scientific tests. Ingredients such as elastins and collagen cannot penetrate and alter your skin. The cosmetics industry is largely unregulated about claims it can make, much to my regret, so there is confusion about what really works. Separating fact from fiction comes with usage and knowledge. In the case of EGF, it is a medically certified fact that it produces physiologically younger skin cells. There is information in the back of this book about how to find RéVive products, the only cosmetics line that contains recombinant human EGF protein.

Over the past twenty years or so, we have become aware of the effects of good diet and exercise on our aging bodies. With the advancements in skin cell regeneration, you will now see that your skin can have extended youth and fitness as well. EGF is not the only new protein that improves the quality of your skin. Laboratories all over the world are working on topical innovations that are equally impressive and promising.

CHAPTER 5

bioengineered cosmetics: what they are and how they work

E GF vastly improves skin without altering the cell structure or skin anatomy. But there are dozens of other growth factors and bioengineered compounds that do alter the skin structure, and some of them even halt or reverse the pace of aging skin. These products are being rigorously tested, and are highly regulated by the federal Food and Drug Administration. Some are currently available although not widely marketed. Others won't hit the market for another couple of years, as they are still in testing phases.

Your skin is composed of many different tissues comprising the dermis and epidermis. The epidermis, the outer layer of skin, is primarily composed of cells called keratinocytes. The deeper layer, the dermis, is primarily made of collagen and elastin, which are connective tissues that provide tensile strength and elasticity. These two are synthesized by cells known as fibroblasts. The dermis and epidermis also contain molecules such as proteoglycans and glycoproteins, held together in a delicate matrix. This matrix acts as mortar, holding together the building blocks that form skin. Aging skin results in these connections breaking down, causing the loss of collagen, proteins, and that youthful matrix. These molecules are relatively large. If you had a handful of collagen or elastin and rubbed it on your skin, it would not penetrate the epidermis. Creams containing collagen or elastin just rest on the surface, making you look smoother only for as long as it remains on your skin, acting as a "filler." The difference with bioengineered topical products is that they focus on changing your skin cell behavior, so that cells produce more collagen and its matrix naturally—to keep the skin's matrix functional and healthy from the inside out, rather than vice versa.

In my research and in other current studies in laboratories around the world, scientists and doctors are developing new ways to protect this delicate matrix of youthful skin. They involve compounds that either change the skin cells directly, change the chromosomes that control skin behavior, or deliver younger human hormones to the skin.

Many of these innovations work because, in one way or another, they restore volume to the face. It has long been my contention that adding volume to the tissues of the face, rather than removing it or pulling it away, is what constitutes the return of youthful looks. These studies into molecularly—even genetically—increasing the production, density, and volume of facial skin, tissue, and bone will bring extraordinary changes to the cosmetic industry in just a few short years.

Protease Inhibitors

Proteases are enzymes released by the epidermis, and are controlled by the hormone levels in your body. There are many types of proteases, and each has a different function, such as holding together skin cells, or sloughing off the dead ones. When these enzymes malfunction or get out of balance, skin diseases result, such as eczema, psoriasis, scleroderma, and dermatitis. One of the proteases is responsible for destroying collagen and elastin, which hold our skin together. As we age, our declining hormone levels prompt this protease to work overtime, breaking down more collagen and elastin, faster than they can be replenished.

Matrix metalloproteinase (MMP) is a specific type of protease. Matrix metalloproteinases are the natural enzymes that are responsible for destroying the healthy matrix of human organs and tissue. When someone has cancer, MMPs go into overdrive, breaking down healthy tissue and spreading tumors. Excessive MMP activity also occurs naturally in aging skin, where it causes wrinkles by destroying our skin's collagen and elastin supplies. Chemical innovations to block MMP activity were originally formulated to help cancer patients. But these compounds have been confirmed to profoundly affect the matrix and collagen network of human skin.

Bioengineered MMP inhibitors (MPI) reproduce the healthy balance of human enzymes and their inhibitors, replacing the off-kilter balance usually found in aging skin. One recently developed MPI product is called MDI Complex, from Atrium Biotechnologies, Inc. This company is using state-of-the-art technology to isolate the molecules in cartilage that inhibit the destructive MMP. Clinical trials have proved the ability of MPI to strengthen the protective function of skin, thereby eliminating redness, fine lines, dark eye circles, and sun spots. It has also proven effective on broken capillaries, spider veins, and even varicose veins on the legs. These maladies were improved by as much as 60 percent in test cases, truly a profound result. Even more impressive, MPIs also proved to strengthen the skin barrier against damage from the sun, warts, moles, injury, and pollutants such as free radicals. MPIs further serve to strengthen the protective function of skin. There is nothing else on the market with such potently beneficial effects on your complexion. This compound is currently available, over the counter, in a topical cream from RéVive called Intensité, as well as Skin Therapy's Advanced B5 Serum with MDI Complex.

Many tests are currently being done on a synthetic MPI called Galardin. It has already been shown to have cancer-preventing qualities. Similarly, Eukaryon Inc., of Massachusetts, has developed two synthetic enzymes that defuse free radicals and their subsequent damage to DNA. These enzymes let the skin cells reproduce for lengthier amounts of time, disproving a long-held belief that it was impossible to extend the lifespan of any organism. These enzymes are still being tested and won't be commercially available before 2006.

Rafaello Laboratories, of California, has taken an expanded approach with MPIs. They have developed not only a topical cream but an oral supplement that contains metalloproteinase inhibitors. Their tests showed that the oral supplement, which contains astaxanthin, omega-3 fatty acids, and glucosamine, penetrated the skin from within the body, while the cream penetrated from the outside. They call this clinically tested system MRT, for matrix rejuvenation technology, and it is now available to consumers (see Resources for more information).

Human Growth Hormone

Human growth hormone (HGH) has proved to reverse many signs of aging, but it also has adverse side effects. Replacing HGH loss with a daily injection of HGH has shown great effects in slowing the aging process by as much as 25 percent. These studies are focusing on HGH's impact on cardiovascular disease and Alzheimer's, but I am closely watching its ancillary effects on aging skin. Many studies have been completed and are currently being reviewed by the Food and Drug Administration. Human growth hormone does have tremendous influence on healthy skin. Since hormones affect far more of your body's systems than the skin, it will be a long time before human growth hormone obtains FDA approval for antiaging, or even as a viable skin care regimen. It is not yet known whether the benefits outweigh the liabilities; be cautious.

Human Growth Factors

Growth factors are not the same as human growth hormone. HGH is a single protein released by the pituitary gland, and it stimulates growth of musculoskeletal tissue. This is the hormone that is absent or greatly diminished in cases of dwarfism. Growth factors are human proteins that influence DNA and stimulate the proliferation of cells and protein synthesis. They are produced locally throughout the body, and not by the pituitary gland. There are thirty-two known growth factors, and some have been used to treat a variety of ailments for the past several years. For example, human growth factors have successfully reestablished normal blood cell production in cancer patients. Some growth factors have proved to be very effective in improving the condition of skin, as you learned about EGF in Chapter 3. But there are others that have only recently been isolated and tested, and they may prove to be the most potent of all.

Another growth factor in the human body is Insulin-like

Growth Factor (IGF). IGF maintains our youthful muscle, bones, and tissue mass. IGF also keeps our blood vessels in good health. It is triggered by hormones naturally produced by our active muscles. As we age, our levels of growth hormone and IGF decline, as do so many things. While injections of HGH and IGF continue to be tested to assess their overall antiaging effects, the topical application of recombinant IGF has been tested on skin, in our own labs. We determined that when IGF was directly applied to the skin, it rejuvenated skin cells faster and with more density. In other words, the skin became thicker, like a young person's skin. The other effect we observed was that IGF helped to maintain the health and volume of the face. As we age, our jawbones get smaller and our muscles atrophy, forcing down the corners of the mouth. The decline in muscle mass and bone mass is estimated at 40 percent between the ages of twenty and eighty. The real loss in volume is due to the decrease in the "mortar" that holds skin together. These are the complex fluids that exist between cell nuclei, collagen bundles, and other components such as proteoglycans, mucopolysaccharides, and peptidoglycans. Their diminution is analogous to letting air out of a balloon—it is one of the primary causes of sagging jowls, nasolabial folds, and other symptoms of the aged face. If you have a photograph of your grandmother at age eighteen, and can compare it to one when she is sixty-five or seventy, chances are the greatest change in her appearance is in the volume of her face.

IGF has been shown to be a pivotal component of tissue repair and muscle tone. Therefore, it not only rejuvenates and thickens facial skin, adding volume, but it also provides nutrients for the underlying tissues of the face.

The topical application of IGF showed such promise (with no

side effects) at transforming postmenopausal skin that it was recently released as a RéVive cream called Intensité. As with all effective topical creams, it takes about eight weeks to see results. But they are quite remarkable.

Kathryn P., a fifty-two-year-old bank executive, had stopped hormone replacement therapy and was feeling well, but she became very depressed. She thought she might feel better if she had a face-lift, so she came to consult me. She really didn't have any excessive furrows or sagging, but she was wrinkled and had a lot of pigment spots from the sun. I urged her to be cautious about the decision, as she might find that aesthetic surgery would not necessarily make her feel better. I encouraged her to seek professional help for clinical depression with a psychiatrist before deciding on surgery. After years of treating patients, I recognize the signs of a person who has more issues than simply how she looks. No one is helped by having facial surgery for the wrong reasons. In the meantime, I prescribed for Kathryn topical creams including Retin-A and IGF. I told her that if she still felt the same way after six months, we could pursue aesthetic surgery.

After three months, I saw Kathryn again and almost didn't recognize her. Her skin was clear and smooth, and even her eyes were brighter. She'd sought counseling and was taking an antidepressant, and she'd used the Retin-A and IGF faithfully. She agreed that she didn't need surgery after all, but still wanted to perk up her appearance. She had a medium peel and continued using the topical creams. She looks terrific and is very happy she did not have surgery.

Paula G. is a fifty-five-year-old high school principal who used IGF in early tests. She had few wrinkles in her African-American complexion, but her skin was dull and mottled. After three months of using IGF cream, her face became smooth and flawless. She loves how it has changed her appearance, and her satisfaction is poured into a renewed energy at work and at home.

Platelet-Derived Growth Factor (PDGF) has been found to have the same healing properties as EGF. It is marketed in a cream from Johnson & Johnson called Regranex, and is used specifically for healing skin ulcers and sores caused by diabetes. In tests, PDGF seemed to have better effects in healing when it was used in conjunction with EGF or IGF. PDGF stimulates the secretion of hyaluronic acid, a natural sugar that keeps skin and muscles healthy. Hyaluronic acid from animals has long been used in moisturizers, and synthetic versions are now being injected into the face instead of collagen and other fillers (see page 106). PDGF is not currently available in a cosmetic application for the skin.

Transforming Growth Factor-beta (TGF-b) has been shown in tests to stimulate DNA synthesis of human skin cells. It heals the skin and also heals the membranes that surround veins, thereby making them less visible. TGF-b stimulates cell repair and heals skin more quickly than other growth factors, and the new skin it produces is often stronger than the old skin. It is still being tested, but has so far proven to be the most powerful of the growth factors. We will have to wait only a couple of years to see TGF-b in skin creams.

In the years since we developed EGF, our labs have been working on cloning a third human growth factor and testing its effects on skin regeneration. This particular human protein is called Keratinocyte Growth Factor (KGF), and it stimulates growth of the lining of the mouth, gums, throat, and epidermis. Research has been completed proving that KGF alleviates the irritating oral side effects of chemotherapy and radiation. From those clinical studies, we learned that KGF (which belongs to a larger group called Fibroblast Growth Factors) was activated by ultraviolet rays. Of course, we all know that UV rays only access the human body through the skin, and we do as much to block them as we can. Sunscreens, vital as they are to our good health, deplete our production of KGF, which is essential for youthful and healthy skin. KGF is the most potent factor in tissue and skin repair, even more than EGF. I jokingly call it EGF on steroids. There are three types of skin cells—the endoderm, which is deep nerve tissue and the lining of organs; the mesoderm, the connective muscle tissue; and ectoderm, which is the outer shell of skin. Where EGF stimulates the cells of all three layers (but primarily the ectodermal), KGF stimulates only the ectodermal cells, delivering a potent boost. KGF has also been shown to increase facial volume in places such as the deep furrows that form from the edges of the lips down to the chin (picture the face of a ventriloquist's dummy). KGF is currently available in a RéVive cosmetic cream called Intensité Volumizing Serum.

There is a cream called Tissue Nutrient Solution (TNS) Recovery Complex from SkinMedica, which contains a mixed fluid extracted from skin cells grown in tissue culture. This hodgepodge solution contains unknown factors, not just known growth factor. It may also contain inhibitory elements that are not known, as it has not been sufficiently analyzed. Only Intensité contains the powerful human proteins needed to actually improve the barrier functions of your skin and add volume to your face.

In our clinical studies, patients such as sixty-year-old Marjorie J. used KGF cream for six months. Marjorie's skin was crepey and almost puckered in her cheek hollows. She used KGF without any other creams such as Retin-A or EGF, but she did use a sunscreen.

Marjorie's skin reacted differently from the way skin reacts to other growth factors: Her skin became thicker and fuller, filling out the fine lines that had covered her cheeks. She could not believe the difference.

Melissa B., a fifty-seven-year-old artist, used KGF for a year, and discovered that her facial skin seemed pinker, thicker, and more "dewy," like it was when she was in her twenties. She then had a medium peel, and found that the KGF helped maintain her new look for four years, twice as long as it might normally have lasted.

KGF not only has powerful local effects on the epidermis, but it has many IGF properties as well. Stimulating KGF receptors on the epidermis causes it to transmit information to the dermis and, in turn, to the subcutaneous layers beneath. This chain reaction is caused by chemical messages and, as a result, it causes the "mortar" fluids to be replenished in the deepest skin layers, bringing a return of youthful volume.

Growth factors have virtually no side effects. We are only on the threshold of accessing their immeasurable benefits.

Transdermal Delivery

Growth factors are relatively large molecules, and effectively delivering proper doses into the body has long been a challenge to scientists. Insulin has the same "size problem." There has yet to be a transdermal patch for delivering insulin, for example, because insulin's molecules are too large. Liposomes were marketed in the 1990s to deliver topical molecules of moisturizers and proteins *through* the skin. They are tiny capsules that hold the active ingredients. But they don't penetrate very far through the epidermis. Newer liposomes called lipoceuticals contain timed-release layers, which allow for extended all-day release of active ingredients, and far deeper penetration of the dermis. This will make lotions such as Retin-A, sunscreens, and moisturizers much more long-lasting.

Nanospheres are the newest microscopic level of topical delivery, minuscule versions of liposomes that can penetrate the skin far more quickly and effectively. This is a cutting-edge breakthrough that will enhance the already amazing effects of growth factors and other bioengineered skin products. Nanospheres are currently available to cosmetics manufacturers, and you will soon start to see them in marketing campaigns for skin creams. But remember: Even with nanospheres, the active ingredient must still be one that has the ability to interact with human skin.

EGF is a relatively large molecule, but it is smaller than collagen, elastin, and liposomes. When new technologies permit more effective delivery of EGF, it will become even more powerful than it currently is. One of the criticisms of cosmetic EGF has been that the molecule is too large to penetrate the dermis. We have performed radioactive dye studies proving that EGF does reach the appropriate target cells, or *stratum germinativum*. The best explanation for this is that there are hundreds of microtraumas in the epidermis that allow enough EGF to penetrate it.

One of the other challenges in formulating new topical solutions is stabilizing the active ingredient—finding ways to maintain the potency after it is in a jar and sitting on a shelf for several weeks, or even longer. The concentration must remain in place once it's been applied to the skin, and remain there long enough to have biochemical effects. Compounds called "spin traps" for skin rejuvenation are currently in testing stages. Spin traps are antioxidants and anti-inflammatories that have the ability to bind free radicals.

As with all topical products, from Retin-A to RéVive, even growth factor compounds need to be used daily for six to eight weeks before you see improvement. But just as damage is cumulative, so is the restoration using human growth factors. After two months, your skin will improve faster and faster, and you will exponentially slow the aging process in your skin.

Our individual aging patterns are related to our genes, which vary widely. We all know some families who "age gracefully," and others who seem to do the opposite. Gerontologists are looking at how we can repair damaged skin by better understanding DNA. There are sixty-one key genes that undergo radical changes between the ages of eight and eighty. Researchers have found that the gene known as SOD1 is the one that fights off free radicals. Another gene controls how quickly we age—it's called Ku80. This gene is controlled by the P53 gene, an important suppressor of tumors that also slows down our organs as we grow old. It seems the body's natural safeguards against cancer are also the ones that cause us to age.

By studying genetic changes, researchers now strongly believe that aging is not a condition where cells simply stop dividing. Aging is a disease where the cells themselves—rather than their division rate—lose quality and integrity.

Great leaps are being made in genetic research as laboratories race to find cures for cancer, Parkinson's, Alzheimer's, and other fatal illnesses. Along the way, doctors such as myself study the findings as they relate to skin behavior. Stem cell research will lead us to the breakthrough wherein we can replace damaged spinal nerves to enable a paraplegic to walk again. And it will also lead to the technology that allows us to simply replace our old skin cells with new ones.

Genetic engineers are now focusing their studies on telomerase, which is the enzyme that protects skin cells from dying. Telomeres are parts of the human chromosome that serve as a "biological clock," shrinking in volume as our natural hormones diminish with age. Telomeres are destroyed not only by aging, but by sun exposure, to the point where our skin cells stop dividing. They are still good cells; they simply stop dividing. Sometimes, defective human telomeres cause skin cancers. To fight back, our bodies produce telomerase, a natural enzyme that counteracts the damaging effects of telomere loss. But, as with most elements, our natural supply of telomerase dries up as we get old. Telomerase has been successfully manufactured in laboratories, and there are studies in the works on telomerase bioengineering at laboratories such as Geron Corporation, among others. Topical application of the bioengineered enzyme stopped the telomeres from shrinking and ceasing cell division. In fact, telomerase prevents aging in at least three kinds of human skin cells. Human skin cells have been rebuilt and revived, over and over again. By 2015, we will see telomerase in topical skin creams with sophisticated delivery systems.

Stem cell research has shown that injecting certain skin cells at regular intervals throughout adulthood can maintain the volume and elasticity of skin. In particular, research on the mesenchymal stem cell (MSC) derived from human tissue has shown that it can repair and prevent the aging of skin. Using cells withdrawn from a patient's own tissue or even bone, injections have shown that these transplanted cells graft and grow onto the impaired structures. There will one day soon be an injection available wherein a patient's skin cells are replenished and restored at regular intervals. Doctors are also studying methods of getting a body's own MSCs (particularly the dense population found in bone marrow) to migrate to areas where they are needed most, for example, the face.

Researchers recently mutated a human gene known as "Indy," which affects our metabolism. This mutation caused DNA to behave as though it were on a calorie-restricted diet. The life span in lab subjects was greatly increased. This is only one of several advances in metabolism studies that merit our attention.

The Magic Pill

As I mentioned in Chapter 2, reducing your calorie intake has been proved to slow the aging process by altering your metabolism. Many people aren't interested in reducing their calories from 2,500 a day, for example, to only 1,300 per day. Some doctors claim that "mesotherapy," "Lipostabil," or collegenase injections can melt pounds away—these cocktails, which include the anesthetic lidocaine, the beta blocker isproterenol, the asthma drug aminophylline, or soy lecithin, have a great list of potential risks and haven't really proved effective. I don't approve of pills such as Phase 2 starch blockers, as they have little effect and do not discourage our unhealthy propensity for eating too much sugar.

Researchers have found chemical compounds that, when taken in pill form, can mimic the physiological effects of eating less. The National Institutes of Health confirmed that a chemical called 4-phenylbutyrate increased the life span of flies by nearly double. Another such compound is known as a CR Mimetic, and it is actively being developed by researchers for human consumption. A compound known as 2-deoxy-D-glucose (2DG) was developed in the 1950s to treat cancerous tumors but, in the 1990s, researchers discovered that this compound also lowered insulin levels. As a result, the human body acted as though it were eating less—hormones became more plentiful, and the body's glucose level was reduced—even though the patient was eating the same amounts of food. The absorption of free radicals was also reduced. Cells seem to go into a protective mode when they are exposed to 2DG, increasing their life span. 2DG is still undergoing clinical trials, and scientists are contending with its apparent risk of toxicity. Although this will prevent it from being marketed for human consumption at the moment, indications are that there might one day be a "magic pill" that mimics lower calorie intake.

The beauty of this genetic research is that it proves the effects of something we already have available to us: a low-calorie diet. Researchers at the University of California at Riverside recently released a study that confirmed that, when older mice were fed a low-calorie diet, *the damage to their genes was reversed.* We will continue to hear about bioengineered landmarks that change the course of aging. But scientists have already established the medical benefits of proper diet for our hearts, our skin, our genes, our longevity. We possess the magic pill already, and you don't even have to pay extra for it. If you want to stay a step ahead of the bioengineers, as well as reverse the damage to your genes, all you need to do is eat less. As you age, a healthy diet should total only about 1,200 calories per day. This is a lot less than most of us currently consume.

CHAPTER 6

step 4: new medical procedures for skin rejuvenation without surgery

As we await the bioengineered topical creams that will repair aging skin cells, there are other treatments currently available to improve your skin's appearance, and the results are remarkable. Some of these are injections, which do nothing more than add volume underneath the skin. Then there is a wide variety of facial peels that can turn back the clock dramatically. As an added benefit, you can have one of these treatments and still use the innovative topical treatments for long-term maintenance of your refreshed new look. Many of these procedures have become accessible and affordable, as witnessed by the growing number of consumers.

Injections

Contrary to what many people believe, removing or tightening parts of the skin structure does not always result in the appearance of youth. *Aesthetic surgery does not re-create youth.* Often it is better to add volume to the face, rather than take it away. Our skin does not bounce back like rubber—when we lose volume in our facial structure, the skin droops and sags. Adding tiny amounts of filler to the facial structure—in the bags under the eyes, perhaps, or to a drooping jowl—often takes years away from your appearance. Most injectables fall into two categories: those that smooth wrinkles, such as Botox, and those that add volume with soft tissue fillers, such as collagen.

BOTOX INJECTIONS

Botox is a trademark for botulinum toxin, and there are similar products known as Myobloc and Dysport. These products block nerve impulses, temporarily paralyzing facial muscles and smoothing wrinkles. More than 850,000 people had such injections in 2001, and that figure more than tripled, to 2.8 million, in 2003. Eighty-six percent of the patients were women, and most were between the ages of thirty-five and fifty.

Botox injections are sometimes offered by salons or aestheticians. As simple and safe as this procedure may be, you should only trust a board-certified medical doctor, such as a dermatologist or plastic surgeon, to perform this procedure. The results remain for only about five months or less, although frequent treatments can increase the length of effectiveness. It is primarily implemented for smoothing forehead lines, crow's feet, eyebrows, and neck creases.

COLLAGEN INJECTIONS

Collagen makes up most of the epidermis—up to 70 percent, in fact. For many years, manufacturers marketed creams containing bovine collagen, claiming that this ingredient would rejuvenate aging skin in humans. Of course, since collagen's molecules are very large (particularly those from a cow), these creams did nothing more than moisturize. Aside from stimulation by human growth factors, nothing is known to restore human collagen, whose natural production virtually grinds to a halt at middle age. However, it was discovered that injections of bovine collagen (also known as Zyderm or Zyplast) served to "fill" lines of the face. There are also injections containing human collagen, such as Cosmoderm and Cosmoplast, which are equally effective and as long-lasting as bovine collagen.

Collagen injections are very safe, although they have more of a risk of allergic reaction than Botox does. Collagen, both bovine and human, also breaks down in less than six months, requiring repeated injections if you want to maintain its effects. These are best for deep lines from the sides of the nose to the mouth (nasolabial folds), or if the corners of your mouth point downward, forming two furrows on either side of the chin. Doctors sometimes call these "puppet mouth" or "marionette" lines. Filler injections also improve certain fatty undereye circles and the "lipstick-bleeding" lip wrinkles called perioral lines.

Hyaluronic acid is a natural sugar found in the human body that is important to the health of your skin. It is an intrinsic component of all living organisms' connective tissues. It has long been used in moisturizers, and is now being used in filler injections. Two new injections that bulk up soft tissues contain hyaluronic acid. Restylane and Perlane are synthetic versions of hyaluronic acid, adding volume to minimize wrinkles in the face. These are effective injections for the jaw line, lips, and nasolabial folds. They also last twice as long as collagen injections, so you need fewer treatments. They are now available in the United States.

In Europe and Canada, hyaluronic acid is derived from rooster combs and marketed under the names Hylaform and Juvederm (it is pending approval in the United States from the FDA). In 2003, many Americans traveled abroad to receive these injections, which last for about a year or two.

Two other soft tissue injections are in use outside of the United States, and are awaiting approval from the FDA here. Artecoll is a largely collagen-derived permanent "micro-implant" that fills facial lines. Radiance (also known as Bioform) is an injectable paste derived from calcium hydroxylapatite, a substance found in bones and teeth. The FDA has currently approved this substance only for those with paralyzed vocal cords and urinary incontinence, but in other countries it has been used to create implants in the chin and cheeks.

There are dozens of other filler-injection materials being used around the world. Some will receive FDA approval and debut in the United States with tremendous marketing campaigns—but don't be hoodwinked. Some of these are fine products, but their implementation and effects are not so different from options we already have.

SILICONE INJECTIONS

Silikon 1000 is a man-made silicone injection that is far more effective than silicone injections of years gone by. Those received horrible publicity, two decades ago, after they were used for breast enhancements, because the injected silicone migrated to other parts of the body. But newer technology and better delivery systems have made silicone a more reliable choice, in certain cases, as a filler injection for the face. Silicone injections are permanent filler material, which distinguishes it from the other options. But silicone still contains the risk of foreign-body reaction.

And, once it is injected into soft tissue, it cannot easily be removed. For safer, permanent results with filler injections, there is another option that is far superior: the autologous fat injection.

The Top Five Nonsurgical Procedures: Number of Patients in the United States in 2003

Botox injection 2,891,390
Chemical peel 995,238
Microdermabrasion 935,984
Laser hair removal 623,297
Collagen injection 576,255

FAT INJECTION

Over the past two decades, doctors have practiced a procedure involving injections of a patient's own fat into parts of the face. There is nothing more natural than one's own tissues to enhance facial aesthetics. The miracle of fat injection is that the effects are often permanent. The newly injected fat (extracted with a needle from the abdomen or thigh) acquires a normal blood supply, and simply becomes an organic part of your face. This procedure is sometimes known as autologous fat transfer. Other injections, except for risky, artificial silicone, are not permanent—they recede in only a matter of months. If performed properly, fat injections last forever.

Fat is also a preferable injection material because it can be used in greater quantity than others, to fill deeper lines of the face. Until recently, however, there was one impediment to the reliability of fat injection. Traditional needles delivered fat in amounts no smaller than a pea, a size that often proved too large to successfully nurture a permanent blood supply. After recent medical innovations, newer injection tools can now provide fat in quantities of micromilliliters, the size of a pinpoint, thereby enabling the healthy establishment of blood supply to the altered areas.

A colleague of mine in New York City, Dr. Sydney Coleman, has refined the instruments for fat injection, and developed a new technique known as LipoStructure. Where liposuction takes fat away, LipoStructure is the transplant of fat from one part of the body to another. Dozens of tiny injections add subtly to the facial structure, until the face is fuller and more youthful. These tiny layers of fat can be injected into the trough under the eyes, the jawline, and even into veiny or bony hands. Fat injection is not a new idea, but the new delivery system has made an extraordinary difference. The photos below provide an example of the effects of LipoStructure.

Another new fat injection technique has been tested by

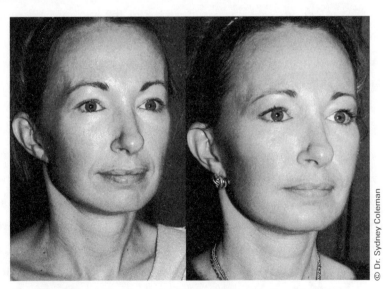

© Dr. Sydney Coleman

A patient before and eighteen months after one LipoStructure® session to her forehead, temples, brow, between eyebrows, nose, eyelids, cheeks, lips, around the mouth, chin, and jawline.

French plastic surgeon Dr. Roger Amar. Fat Autograft Muscle Injection (FAMI) is based on the fact that the volume lost with aging is not only fat, but muscle and bone as well. Dr. Amar based his technique on the fact that transplanted fat is more likely to survive permanently if it is placed against a muscle. These fat injections go directly into the muscles of facial expression. This works exceedingly well for those patients who have hollowed eye circles or flattened cheeks, nasolabial folds, or receding chin and lips. He has even found success using this method on patients who have already had a face-lift and don't want the pulled skin of multiple surgeries.

Transconjunctival Deep Lipotransfer (TDL) is another licensed term for a fat injection procedure. This one addresses undereye bags by adding fat deep within the lower eyelid muscle, instead of taking fat away, as is usually done. TDL recontours the lower eyelid, and the fat stays in place underneath the muscle.

Fat injections are a marvelous option for patients of color. Since there are no scarring or pigment risks, injections can eliminate furrows and wrinkles for Asians, Hispanics, and African Americans.

TISSUE IMPLANTS

There are now surgical compounds known as AlloDerm and Fascian that are used in facial implants. They are derived from the fascia, or dermis, of human cadavers. They do not last as long as collagen injection, but they indicate that there will be more progress in the near future on effective and organic filler materials. Isolagen is the name for the injection compound that is derived from one's own skin cells after a small amount has been excised by needle biopsy and cultured in laboratory test tubes. After a few weeks, the patient's own fibroblasts have multiplied, and this compound is injected into parts of the face. The goal is that the higher quantity of fibroblasts will increase the natural production of collagen. But there is no evidence that this process actually occurs. Isolagen requires multiple insertions over the course of six months, and it can take that long to notice any results. These are not as dramatic or as long-lasting as LipoStructure using fat injections. One day, there may be better ways to use human tissue and fibroblasts.

There are a variety of facial implants that are relatively noninvasive. Advanta and UltraSoft lip implants, for example, are easily inserted through the mouth—these offer a more defined lip border and are not as "poofy" as injectables. But I think, for now, fat injection is still the superior option.

Injectables such as Isolagen, Dermologen, and Alloderm are simply temporary fixes that are little improvement over collagen injections and are more costly. The one truly effective filler is autologous fat, which is fat from your own body.

Chemical Peels

Peels, laser treatments, and dermabrasion perform the same purpose—they cause controlled injury to the surface of the skin, so that the healthier, deeper cells surface while they are still fresh. Peels essentially hasten the process of skin replenishment, and the degree of improvement is determined by how deep each treatment is. The deeper the treatment, the more noticeable are the results—the skin is smoother and obtains a healthy glow. Blotchy skin becomes cleaner and clearer, acne scars fade, and your natural collagen production is stimulated. Peels essentially do the same thing as topical creams such as Retin-A or AHA— sloughing the surface skin cells—but they act more swiftly and often more deeply. The results are instant, and they are long-lasting.

Peels come from various sources—from fruit acid and glycolic acid compounds (like AHA creams) or chemical compounds such as trichloroacetic acid (TCA). Regardless of the source, their basic actions are similar, and results are determined by the strength of the compound. It is a fact that a patient who starts using Retin-A and hydroquinone six weeks prior to a peel will recover more quickly and have more dramatic results.

A *micro peel* uses a 30 to 50 percent glycolic solution and can be applied by a trained skin care technician. This is also called a "very superficial" peel, and it works extremely well on acne-prone skin, helping to erase dark spots and fine lines. After a micro peel, the skin will slough imperceptibly for a couple of weeks, resulting in a glowing complexion. For best effects, a patient should have this peel done four times over the course of three months, and then once every three months thereafter.

A *superficial peel* is a slightly stronger version of a micro peel. The same chemicals are used, only in higher concentrations. The sloughing of skin will continue for a couple of days, so many people call this a "weekend peel." For best results, most doctors prescribe one per month for six months, and then every other month thereafter. The solutions might include glycolic acid, salicylic acid, resorcinol, or a combination known as Jessner's solution.

Both micro peels and superficial peels are safe and relatively affordable. They are perfect for patients who want better skin without spending thousands of dollars and weeks of recovery time. With follow-up treatments, these peels will remove fine lines and blotchy skin.

There are stronger peels, however, that produce quite dramatic results: medium chemical peels, deep peels, laser peels, and dermabrasion. Sometimes these treatments need to be repeated once or twice to achieve the desired effects. These procedures must be implemented by a board-certified physician, preferably a plastic surgeon or dermatologist.

For a *medium chemical peel*, the compounds used are the same as those for a micro peel, such as TCA or glycolic acid, only in stronger concentrations. Your doctor might give you a sedative, as these stronger peels cause more intense burns on the face in order to destroy old skin cells. A burning sensation lasts about five minutes, and then a neutralizing agent is applied to stop the action. The skin remains red for several days after a medium peel. In the course of a week, the skin flakes off and reveals a brighter, youthful complexion. It's like a snake shedding its skin. A medium peel will soften deep facial lines, and eliminate brown spots and acne. They are particularly effective, as all peels are, on fairer skin. Olive skin and darker skin tones have a slightly higher risk of hyperpigmentation or hypopigmentation as a result of a peel, but a medical professional knows how to forestall these risks. The cost is around $3,000, and the effects last for a couple of years. Many women choose a regimen of having a medium peel every other year, and it makes them feel terrific. TCA peels can also be applied sparingly to the neck and hands. Patients should be aware that their skin might even look worse for a few days, while the skin exfoliates.

Another variation of this procedure is the Obagi Blue Peel, which combines TCA with tretinoin and hydroquinone. The effects will last up to two years, although many patients choose to repeat one every year. These peels are enhanced if you begin using Obagi cream, or Retin-A and hydroquinone, about six weeks before the procedure. These topical creams will actually increase the effects of the peel, as well as speed your healing. The only problem is that extended use of these products can cause redness and constant inflammation.

Joe G., a fifty-one-year-old corporate executive, had a TCA peel on his face, neck, and hands. He had a lot of sun damage and old, shallow acne scars. After the treatment, he had no scars at all, and the sun damage had been reversed. We started him on a KGF topical regimen, which permitted him sun exposure (unlike Retin-A), and now he feels more motivated to play racquetball and keep in shape. His renewed energy helped him lose ten pounds and focus on his work, as well as his recharged marriage. His wife was thrilled and opted to have the same procedure herself!

A deeper chemical procedure, a *phenol peel,* is performed under sedation and takes nearly an hour. Because one's heart rhythms must be monitored under sedation, this procedure usually requires a hospital visit—it is not an "in-office" procedure. The phenol solution deeply penetrates the skin to remove all wrinkles and freckles, and it even tightens skin. Phenol removes acne scars, lip lines, and dark pigments. The effects last for years. Although they may be performed on olive-toned skin, these peels are best for people with fair skin without too many freckles, so the demarcation lines are not apparent. Some doctors claim that patients who get a phenol peel reduce their risk of developing skin cancer in the future. I don't think I would go that far, but it would make sense since this peel erases any traces of existing sun damage. Recovery takes at least ten days, although the skin may remain red for as long as two months.

If you are fair and heavily freckled, it will eliminate all the freckles on your face, which may not look natural if your neck and hands are still freckled. There may even be a "line" where the freckles stop. Phenol may not be used on any other part of the body, including the neck, because it leaves a line of color demarcation. However, one phenol peel can last a lifetime. Even though some doctors perform this procedure on olive-skinned individuals, I think it should only be performed on patients with fair skin. The risk of pigment demarcation is too high for darker-skinned patients.

Dermabrasion

Dermabrasion uses a mechanical device that is not unlike a sanding machine, and is performed under sedation. It's been around for years and still gives good results, particularly for broad and deep acne scars and lip lines. It is not as effective as a phenol peel, and may require several visits to the doctor. With all the newer techniques available, especially lasers, dermabrasion has taken a real backseat. However, I still think for certain people with acne, it is great. The effects don't last as long as with phenol either—about two to four years. But with the advent of lasers, dermabrasion is used less and less frequently.

Microdermabrasion is an unrelated and far less invasive sloughing treatment. Aluminum oxide crystals in a little vacuum tube slough off dead skin in a matter of minutes. Microdermabrasion is also known as Diamond Peel, Dermapeel, or Parisian peel—all of them different marketing terms for the same thing. These are quite inexpensive and show instant, if marginal results. Multiple treatments every few weeks yield better results, particularly when used in conjunction with Retin-A or a sophisticated topical regimen.

82% women   83% Caucasian

18% men   6% Hispanic

             5% African American

             3% Asian American

             3% other

Laser Peels

Another example of breaking technology is the advanced precision of lasers and tiny surgical scopes for procedures that once required scalpels, incisions, and scars. "Laser" is actually an acronym for Light Amplification by Stimulated Emission of Radiation. This amplified light beam is so strong it can cut a diamond. Laser peels work well on lip lines, age spots, rosacea, broken blood vessels, wrinkles, small moles, and acne scars. This treatment is sometimes also called laser resurfacing, lasabrasion, or laser peeling, and it is quite expensive—$5,000 or higher.

Instead of using chemicals to burn off the outer layer of skin, laser peels use beams of light to vaporize the skin in a controlled area. It also "shrinks" the new skin on your face. Just like chemical peels, depths and recovery periods vary with the strength of the procedure. Results last anywhere from two to ten years.

Lasers are superb for people who want to eliminate large freckles or deep age spots, melasma from pregnancy, or rosacea. Lasers can target specific areas with deeper treatment, and can be used on the face, hands, neck, or any area of the body.

Erbium laser treatments are the equivalent of a medium

peel—not too invasive, but providing excellent results. This laser treatment takes only twenty minutes, and may be redone after five years.

Lighter laser treatments include the Q-switch ruby, Alexandrite, and Erbium: YAG lasers. The optimum laser is selected based on which pigment color is being lightened (e.g., a yellow tone, a brown spot, a red scar). A vascular laser can spot-repair rosacea, red birthmarks, and broken blood vessels.

The strongest laser is the ultrapulsed carbon dioxide (CO_2) laser. Many doctors now use the newer technology of intense pulse light (IPL), such as the Quaddra Q4. This uses more wavelengths of light than regular lasers. The equipment depends on which one your doctor prefers to use. The effects of IPL are equivalent to those from CO_2 laser peels, except IPL needs to be repeated about four times over six months.

The ultrapulsed CO_2 laser has the most effects on all wrinkles and sun damage, although it takes a few more weeks of recovery and has more potential complications. The skin is oozy and red for a good ten days, then dark pink for a couple more weeks. A CO_2 peel is the laser equivalent of a deep chemical peel. CO_2 also enhances the performance of your skin's collagen, improving skin tone as it erases wrinkles. The procedure virtually "shrink-wraps" the face so, in addition to losing the wrinkles, many of the effects of gravity are improved as well. Often, patients look better than if they'd had a major face-lift; however, it is not to be taken lightly.

Among laser peels, this one requires a lot of recovery time, so I only recommend it in extreme cases, such as when a patient has severe "cobwebs" of wrinkles all over his face. Of all the procedures I have performed, patients unanimously agree that this one

(CO$_2$ laser resurfacing) requires the most arduous and painful recovery. The scars are red and weepy for a couple of weeks, and it may take as long as six months for the redness to go away. Patients describe it as feeling as though they have dried soap on their faces. But, for the right patient—a fair-haired, sun-damaged, markedly wrinkled person—CO$_2$ laser resurfacing can be remarkable.

PhotoDynamic Therapy (PDT) is a laser treatment that is enhanced by a light-sensitizing solution applied to the skin prior to the laser or pulsed light. It works very well on acne, scars, rosacea, and blotchy skin. Because the results are magnified, fewer treatments may be required.

For those with olive-toned or brown skin, the new lasers are far safer than chemical peels. There is a much smaller risk of pigment loss, particularly with the nonablative lasers such as the variable-pulsed KTP laser, and Photomodulation, which uses low-level, nonthermal light energy. Photorejuvenation uses short pulses of light that do not injure the epidermis. In addition there are new nonablative "lasers," such as those that use radio frequency heat instead of intense light.

Radio Frequency (RF) Ablation

Radio frequency ablations are nonlaser peels that use radio frequency devices to tighten and lift the skin, such as Thermage ThermaCool TC and Thermalift. Heat and radio waves pass through the skin and encourage collagen production, while tightening skin and removing wrinkles along the way. At the same time, a cooling spray protects the skin from scarring. Deep structures tighten immediately. After just one treatment, some patients have a 50 percent tightening in folds, such as those on the forehead, eyelids, jowls, and neck. It takes about ten minutes, costs about $2,000, and there is virtually no recovery time. After six months, the full effects of rejuvenated collagen bring an even more pronounced glow to the face. Some doctors also use it on the abdominal skin and sagging arms. It may prove to be a great treatment to include with a liposuction, which doesn't contract skin once fat has been removed. According to the manufacturers, the results last up to two years, although I have observed it to last about one year, in most cases.

Beverly R., a sixty-five-year-old African-American singer, had a lot of wrinkles—not any freckles or scars, but a fine network of lines on her cheeks, chin, neck, and forehead. I felt that her skin was too dark for a CO_2 laser peel. Instead, she had a Thermalift peel. All of her wrinkles simply vanished. Her friends wondered if she'd had a face-lift, but all she had was a simple nonsurgical peel.

These results are preliminary. Many times new procedures are heavily promoted by the manufacturers of the mechanical systems. I am an extremely conservative surgeon, and I feel that new procedures such as RF ablation need at least five years in the marketplace before you seriously consider them. I never jump on a bandwagon to offer the newest procedure, nor should you as a prospective patient. The thousands of pages of marketing materials I regularly receive from manufacturers only show preliminary successes. All procedures carry risks, and these are almost never presented in the sales materials.

Whether you opt for a laser peel or a chemical peel, most doctors will complement the treatment with a topical regimen using Retin-A or the other creams I recommend. Peels give you a "jump start" on a fresher complexion, and they can last for many years with the support of a topical regimen.

Any of these procedures may work for you. You need to consider cost, recovery time, and risk. Also important is how much improvement you seek to achieve. Obviously, the more improvement you desire, the greater the cost and the recovery process. It is not something to be considered lightly. Shop around for several doctors, get information off the Internet (websites are listed in the back of this book), and talk to patients of the doctors you are consulting. Remember: It is not as simple as going to a hair salon, contrary to what beauty magazines may have you believe.

If you have fair skin, chemical peels are as safe and effective as laser peels. The cost is equivalent, and a trained medical professional can guide you through the process with which he or she is most familiar. If you want to improve specific spots, laser may be more efficient than a chemical peel. For those with darker skin tones, I would definitely recommend laser over a chemical peel. They are widely available and immensely effective in rejuvenating your complexion. One day, the precision of pulsed light and non-ablative lasers will displace the chemical peel altogether. But both remain very helpful to those with fairer skin.

Don't Forget the Dentist

The condition of your teeth significantly reflects your age, so don't forget to accompany your facial enhancements with white, shining teeth. Your dentist has dozens of options for improving your smile. There are many instant whiteners that make an enormous difference to your appearance. Dentists are also getting into the "nonsurgical face-lift" arena with a new prosthetic implant that helps eliminate wrinkles around the mouth, lips, chin, and cheek. I would be wary of these until they are more widely used. Custom-fitted dental implants from Medical Matrix displace the lost volume from our receding gums and jawbones. It's called Angel Lift—a removable implant—and it is now being disseminated to dentists throughout the United States. Of course, replacing lost rear teeth can also realign your jaw.

Many patients are now getting porcelain veneers on their front teeth. This can actually serve to push your lips slightly forward, making them appear fuller.

CHAPTER 7

the 4-step overview

A cross the United States, you should have regional access to all of the treatments described in this book. The Resources section at the back of this book also provides contacts for finding qualified doctors for each procedure. Much of what should determine both your nonsurgical and surgical aesthetic options is based on where you are in life. There are exceptions, of course, but my skin care philosophy includes general guidelines based on your age. A twenty-year-old would not benefit from the same treatments prescribed to a seventy-year-old. The procedure you choose should depend on many factors: how much available recovery time you have, how much you want to spend, and so forth. If you want tighter skin all over, laser might be what you should choose. But if you have only five days off work to recover, a lighter peel might be better. Don't choose the latest technology simply because it's getting lots of press or it worked for your friend. Think about what you want to fix, and find the doctor who understands what it is you seek to achieve.

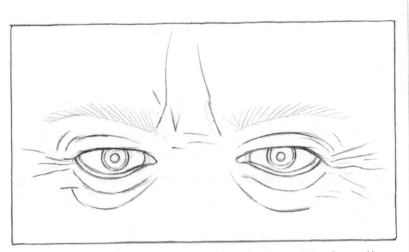

crow's-feet, puffy eyelid, droopy eyelid, undereye circles, furrowed brows

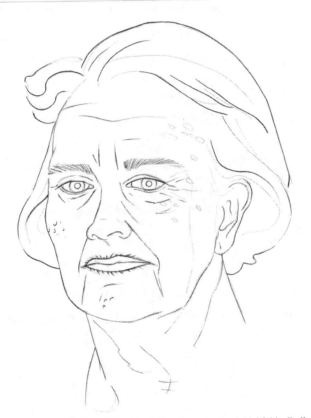

sagging jowls, lines in forehead, lines in neck, nasolabial folds, lip lines, marionette lines, age spots, acne scars, deep cheek lines

ADVANCED PROCEDURES AT A GLANCE

Treatment	Good For
Laser peel	Acne, rosacea, fine lines, moles, lip lines, sagging jowls, crow's-feet, dilated blood vessels, wrinkles, veins in hands, collagen rejuvenation; dark and light skin
Chemical peel	Fair-skinned patients with fine lines, wrinkles, lip lines, age spots, and blemishes
Dermabrasion	Fair-skinned patients with deep lines, acne scars, lip lines, precancerous growths, periorbital lines
RF ablation	Dark- or light-skinned patients with wrinkles, sagging jowls, droopy neck; collagen rejuvenator
Sclerotherapy	Spider veins
Fat injection and filler injection	Undereye circles, sagging jowls, nasolabial folds, marionette lines, droopy neck, lip lines, forehead lines, deep creases
Botox injection	Frown lines, crow's-feet, forehead creases, neck creases
Retin-A and RéVive with EGF, KGF, or IGF	Mottled skin, age spots, acne, crow's feet, lip lines, fine lines, sun damage, smokers' skin, loss of facial volume
RéVive with MPI (such as Sans Veines or Intensité)	Undereye circles, broken blood vessels and capillaries on face and hands, spider veins

The following chapters will guide you toward the treatments most appropriate for you, for now and for the rest of your life.

customize the

program to your age

and to the season

CHAPTER 8

under 35: stay younger longer

A s clichéd as it sounds, our skin starts aging from the moment we are born. But when you're in your twenties and thirties, your skin appears to be in its prime. The levels of collagen, elastin, and human proteins are healthy and balanced. Your muscle tone and skin elasticity are strong. The sagging and drooping caused by gravity and volume loss are still some years away. But this is the time when what you do and don't do for your complexion will later reveal itself during your forties and fifties. During this key period, a lot can be done to prevent the aging of your skin later on in life. This is the time to ensure your future healthy skin, and to take actions to maintain its vitality.

Patients in their twenties and early thirties do not really need special facial treatments or procedures other than a moisturizer and sunscreen, or perhaps acne treatment. Even if you have oily or darker skin, you still need a moisturizer and sunscreen. Choosing the best products for you, however, can be daunting. There is no hard-and-fast rule about what brands you should use. Just as each of our fingerprints is completely distinctive, the composition of our skin is equally unique. Everyone's skin is composed differently, with varying levels of collagen, elastin, proteins, oils, acids, water, and melanin, in a combination that also determines the thickness of your skin. Because of these billions of variations, no single skin cream is going to be the perfect one for all of us. The only products anyone can tell you to use are the ones you've tried yourself.

My friend Sandi S., thirty-nine, swears that Murad is the only product she can use on her face. Her skin is flawless, and she is a walking advertisement for Murad. But my patient Judith, thirty-two, called Murad a waste of money. After using this product (primarily composed of plant extracts), Judith broke out with pimples for the first time in fifteen years. She then tried the oil-free version, and the same thing happened. This treatment simply wasn't appropriate for her skin. That is true for every cleanser and skin cream: Some of them may cause an irritating reaction with your particular skin dynamic.

We still must resort to old-fashioned trial and error in order to identify the best products for ourselves. And, chances are, the one that works for you may not be the same product that works so well for your coworker or even your sister. Finding the right product can be time-consuming and expensive. I recommend certain cleansers and creams in this book because I have found them to be the least irritating and most effective for the broadest range of patients. However, even these might react poorly to your skin. Shop around, and try others. When you find the one that works for you, stick with it! If you are still dissatisfied, visit a dermatologist, who can use medical supervision to direct you to the proper daily treatments.

After finally finding cleansers and creams that bring the optimum condition to your complexion, you may observe subtle changes after a couple of years. That's because your skin is always evolving. During your childbearing years, you experience more metabolite buildup, sun and free-radical exposure, and simple aging, causing the delicate matrix of your skin to change. You may find that after one or two years, your tried-and-true skin care regimen isn't working anymore. It is not uncommon to begin the search all over again. But as time passes, better products are created anyway. You should expect to alter or add to your regimen every couple of years, perhaps for the rest of your life. As you age, more demands will be made on your skin care regimen. Gone are the days when Pond's cold cream sufficed for a lifetime.

I am a great proponent of alternating skin care treatments. However, if your skin looks fine, maintain your regimen for as long as you like. But if your skin starts to react differently, look for a change. Your skin needs a break from time to time. I recommend choosing two different products, containing different ingredients, and alternating them every six months. For example, long-term daily use of an AHA cream or Retin-A is not the best regimen for your skin. Our skin sometimes builds up a resistance to the constant use of a single active ingredient. Think of it this way: Your body wouldn't maintain its optimal condition if all you ate was spinach or broccoli for an entire year, even though these are healthy foods. Like the rest of your body, your skin needs variation in nutrients to maintain its optimal health. Aging is caused by so many variables that decrease the regenerative power of skin and reduce facial volume. It is difficult to pinpoint a particular pill or cream that slows the process for everyone across the board.

The only extra skin treatments you might need in your twenties are mild facial peels, which can reduce freckles as well as acne. If you become pregnant, you may get dark pigment spots on your face. These are called *melasma,* and are caused by hormonal changes due to pregnancy or using birth control. Dark spots caused by the sun, or "liver spots," are technically called *lentigenes.* Melasma and lentigenes are alleviated by mild peels, as well as topical creams such as hydroquinone and Retin-A. Microdermabrasion is also very helpful to a younger patient who wants to even out his skin tone.

Janice A., a twenty-five-year-old violinist, was very self-conscious about her acne scars and a dark birthmark on her cheekbone, under her right eye. After a series of microdermabrasion treatments and topical hydroquinone, her skin became much smoother, and the dark spot faded significantly. I also advised her to add sunscreen to her moisturizer, so the sun wouldn't bring back the dark pigment of her birthmark. She chose an oil-free sunscreen so it wouldn't cause additional acne. Her skin became positively glowing, and her renewed confidence was reflected in her musical performance.

People currently in this age group will one day benefit from amazing bioengineered skin care products that are now in development. Ten or twenty years from now, such products will enable you to look younger far longer than your parents did. But at this time of life, it is not absolutely necessary to use expensive bioengineered products. I don't usually recommend EGF until a patient is around thirty, because she simply doesn't show the signs of aging until then. If you are only in your twenties, EGF would still benefit your skin, but it would be difficult to notice a visible difference. There is not yet established proof that EGF can have an effect prior to actual symptoms of aging. Not so with microdermabrasion or a fruit acid peel—those results are quite visible. If you're in your twenties or thirties, you need not "turn back the clock." However, careful treatment—sunscreen, mild peels, and such—helps you slow down the clock by as much as ten years.

It is not too soon for you to map out an aesthetic program now, to plan for the future. Your family's genetic history definitely indicates your susceptibility to skin cancer, wrinkles, and sagging. You can make a huge difference by minimizing your exposure to sunlight, stopping smoking, and drinking less alcohol. Life can still be fun without these elements! Revel in the fact that you will remain youthful far longer without them.

Birth and Birth Control

Many patients in their twenties and thirties take birth control medications, and these can affect your complexion as well. If you take birth control and start suffering from acne, ask your doctor about switching to another kind of pill. Keep trying new ones until you find the one that does not cause your face to break out.

If you are pregnant, the body's hormones can cause dark pigment spots, but it is better to wait until after you give birth before treating these. Pregnancy brings on a fluctuation in hormones, less physical activity, and weight gain, which also affect the overall tone of your skin. If you know you won't be having more children, you might choose to have laser treatments to decrease your stretch marks as well as the pigment spots on your face. Consult your doctor, but not until you have decided not to be pregnant again. Renewing your exercise routine will also bring back a glow to your complexion.

The Miracle Treatment

You can moisturize and get peels during these youthful years, but the most important thing to remember is this: Do no harm. In addition to sun protection and not smoking, a healthy diet and exercise play the most vital role in the long-term evolution of your complexion. Avoiding sugars and unhealthy fats can keep you lean for a lifetime. The oxygen surge provided by exercise can continuously revitalize your skin. Proper eating and regular exercise can reverse the aging of your cells, inside and out. You are in your prime now but, even better, you are also at the stage in life when you can delay the signs of aging by as much as ten or twenty years, if you work at it. You may not have a need for the miracle creams at this age, but you possess a far more powerful tool in shaping your face of the future. This tool is your personal combination of lifestyle choices.

Remember: Aesthetic surgery cannot re-create youth.

Eat Right and Dance as Often as Possible

Use a healthy body to keep your skin young. Avoid processed foods, sugars, and fats and get into the habit of drinking water wherever you go. When you go out to eat in a restaurant or at a friend's house, request water instead of soda or tea. It doesn't need to be bottled water!

When your body is inadequately hydrated, a whole series of

biochemical and metabolic changes occur—many of the biochemical reactions in your body trigger hormones designed to preserve water. This takes even more energy and accelerates the aging process.

Alice K. is a forty-six-year-old sales rep who has the clearest, peachiest, most translucent skin I have ever seen. Unlike her mother and her sister, she looks nearly twenty years younger than she is. Without extraordinary genes and excessive skin treatments, she attributes her beautiful skin to the fact that she has been guzzling water since she was a teenager. Her friends always teased her about it, but Alice provided her skin with such an abundance of oxygen that now, in middle age, she has an exceptionally youthful complexion. She is proof that water is indeed the fountain of youth.

Maintaining a budding career or raising young children keeps you active, but not in a dedicated, stress-relieving manner. Start a regimen of walking, running, yoga, Jazzercise, swimming, or Pilates, or a combination thereof, at least twice a week. Lifting two-pound or five-pound hand weights is also superb for good conditioning. It is important enough for you to make time for it, no matter how busy you are. Look for shortcuts, if you must—ten minutes of stair-climbing, for example, has the cardiovascular effect of thirty-six minutes of walking. Park at the very end of the parking lot when you go shopping, so you must walk more.

Get in the habit of making an appointment with yourself to work out a little each week. If you don't schedule the time, something else will absorb that hour without your even knowing it. Theresa E., a thirty-two-year-old real estate agent, has dozens of appointments on a daily basis. And every Tuesday and Thursday, she has a four o'clock appointment to attend yoga class. This is as important to her as any other meeting all week. Writing this in her datebook prevents her from scheduling something else at those times.

Finding time to work out is like finding time for our spiritual lives—if we don't aggressively make the time, it won't happen. If I don't make myself go to church (perhaps for you it is meditation, or volunteer work, or a 12-step program), I know my spiritual health will deteriorate. Poor skin is a direct reflection of the state of our bodies. There is no hard science behind this statement, of course. But I have spent many years closely observing my own habits and those of other people. I truly believe our skin and exterior reflect our degree of spirituality. Our spiritual condition is like building a muscle—it requires exercise and repetition.

The Exceptions for Aesthetic Surgery in Your Prime

I believe that a patient in her twenties or thirties should have an antiaging aesthetic procedure on the face only in exceptional circumstances. I see many women of this age, however, who want breast enhancement, a nose revision, or liposuction on their thighs and hips. These structural changes can go a long way toward improving self-esteem, and they are relatively safe procedures.

Mary L., a twenty-six-year-old bank secretary, came to see me about a breast enhancement. She had been self-conscious about her size A breasts for a decade. She was very pretty and outgoing, but she always felt that her clothes didn't fit her properly. She wanted a little self-confidence to help her in the dating world, and had finally saved enough money for breast implants. After the surgical procedure, she was thrilled with her new figure. I support women who want to make this change while in their twenties— they're old enough to know it is important to them, and young enough to eliminate years of self-consciousness and discomfort. I've seen women become virtually reborn after a breast augmentation, leading more productive lives and finding new happiness in all areas of life. Our appearance is important to our psyche.

Marla Z., thirty-two, was a patient who wanted her breasts reduced in size. She had two young children and was suffering from terrible backaches.

"I feel as though I'm seventy years old," she told me. "There was once a time when I liked having size DD breasts, but now I feel like they're simply excess baggage. They make me look like a saggy grandmother."

When we completed the breast reduction procedure, Marla felt rejuvenated. Her back pain disappeared, and she was able to keep up with her kids. Some women deliberate about this procedure for decades and, when they finally do it, they wish they'd done it years earlier. Large breasts on a thin young woman can make her appear overweight and matronly. These situations are perfect for aesthetic surgery while you are still relatively young.

Another good example of beneficial surgery for a younger patient is rhinoplasty—a nose job. So many men and women suffer through their teens and twenties concerned about their appearance. Nothing is as satisfying as seeing a patient reborn with a new nose. You can certainly have this procedure done later in life, but why wait? If it bothers you, consult a plastic surgeon about having your nose refined. I could not wait until I graduated high school at nineteen: I immediately had a rhinoplasty. This is something you shouldn't hesitate to do—it is completely safe and almost always extremely successful.

I also encourage patients who would like their ears reshaped—otoplasty—to do this at an early age. This is a common procedure for young men as well as women. I frequently perform this procedure on children as young as eight years old, whose ears may stick out away from the head. After otoplasty, young ears grow normally but they are now flat against the skull.

Another good candidate for early procedures is a patient who has acne or deep scars from acne. Dermabrasion and laser treatments can make your skin much smoother and easier to clean and keep healthy.

All of these surgical procedures are safe and provide long-lasting results. If these particular conditions are bothersome to you, take care of them with the help of a good surgeon.

MOST PERFORMED AESTHETIC SURGICAL PROCEDURES IN 2003 FOR PATIENTS AGED 19–34

as reported by the American Society for Aesthetic Plastic Surgery

Nose reshaping	141,944
Breast augmentation	114,005
Liposuction	90,575
Tummy tuck	20,232
Breast lift	15,209
Eyelid surgery	10,658

The number of patients undergoing liposuction, breast enhancement, and breast reduction has nearly tripled since 1997. The largest age group represented in these procedures are those between nineteen and thirty-four, and each patient spent anywhere from $3,000 to $6,000 for the procedure. Interestingly, in my practice, most of these patients have modest incomes, earning less than $50,000 per year.

Should a patient in this age group have a face-lift? Absolutely not. The muscles and skin are still in prime condition.

Surgery would only alter natural features. The only major facial procedure I would recommend is a medium TCA peel, laser treatment, or dermabrasion for someone who had significant acne scarring that was not helped by microdermabrasion. Acne marks can become deeper with age. Once upon a time, insurance companies used to pay for this treatment, but not anymore.

Your natural facial features are really beautiful during this time of your life. If you find yourself dissatisfied with how you look, and your skin condition is good, visit a salon for a makeover. Professional cosmetologists can show you how to accent your best features using simple makeup techniques and hairstyling. Any man or woman in his or her twenties can be made to look extraordinarily beautiful, without any medical treatment at all. It is my experience that most younger patients underestimate the impact of properly applied makeup and hairstyling.

The Routine for Your Twenties and Thirties

DAILY

> Cleanse with mild soap
> Tone with moisturizer
> Protect with sunscreen

BIWEEKLY

> Exfoliate with AHA acid, two or three times per week

ANNUALLY

> Professional microdermabrasion or fruit acid peel every
>> three months, or as needed
> Visit dermatologist for skin cancer prevention

This is the critical age where proper skin care will pay off for the rest of your life. It's easy to believe that sunscreen is not important during your younger years, but in fact, the opposite is true. You can't take back your sun exposure, and the damage accumulates over the years. Youth is your key asset—and youth, above all, is what all my patients most desire. I have never seen a twenty-five-year-old who is not beautiful. We can make certain facial parts look better, such as removing bags under the eyes, but no surgery can re-create that fluid-filled skin you see under the eyes of a younger person. When you have youth, maximize it through makeup, styling, and preventative skin maintenance. As I said before, it is a known fact that surgery cannot re-create youth.

Get a Tan

Some patients tell me they love their wrinkle-free complexions but, at times, they still yearn for the youthful appearance of a suntan. Many have tried self-tanning lotions, which use a chemical called dihydroxyacetone to turn skin brown. Self-tanning creams are non-toxic and far safer than actual sun exposure or tanning booths, both of which can cause skin cancer. And self-tanning "spray booths" have made the application more effective. If you'd like a pick-me-up in the middle of the summer, go ahead and try a topical tanning treatment at a salon. Or try a self-tanning cream such as Neutrogena Build-A-Tan, among many new brands available at retailers.

Be aware that if you have any dark pigment spots, the self-tanning creams will significantly darken those as well. Sometimes, a simple body makeup or foundation can add color instead. New products look very natural, and many provide sunscreen coverage as well. There are creams and pressed powders, and many are oil-free and hypoallergenic. Look for makeup with a tone just one or two shades darker than your natural skin color. Good product lines include MAC, Neutrogena, Aveda, L'Oréal, Ultima II, Prescriptives, and Revlon.

Just seeing yourself with a tan for the first time in years will make you feel terrific! There is actually a biological reason why we like suntanned skin. It makes the contour of our body more visible to others, enhancing the shapes of our muscles. A fair-skinned man won't necessarily show his washboard abs, even if he has them. Add a tan or some makeup, however, and they will magically appear.

CHAPTER 9

from 36 to 55: cosmetic care now, current procedures that really work, and new products on the way

Most of us know that when we hit our mid-forties, the signs of aging skin are everywhere on our bodies. You have dark spots on your face, hands, arms, and chest, partly due to hormonal changes but largely due to years of intermittent sun exposure. You have much drier skin, due to a natural decline in hormones. The dermis, which is 70 percent collagen, loses mass and volume as your natural collagen levels decline. This brings on fine lines on your face and hands. Years of smiling and frowning have formed dynamic wrinkles near your mouth and eyes. Your muscles and bones are no longer as strong and vibrant as they once were, so the underlying structure of your face is not as voluminous, particularly near the jawline. Gravity is taking its toll too—sagging occurs at the eyes, jowls, or neck. This is caused by the loss of the intercellular matrix that holds our skin together. Even your hair is not the same—it is lighter in color and texture. For men, and even most women, the hairline starts receding.

Sounds dreadful, doesn't it? It happens to all of us, however. And, in this age, we now have many treatments that can actually reverse the damage. In the last decade, aesthetic surgical procedures in the United States have increased more than 1,000 percent, from roughly 100,000 per year to 1,600,000. In that time, the number of plastic surgeons in this country has tripled. However, I am a firm believer that not everyone should have aesthetic surgery.

Just over a year ago, I met a forty-year-old woman named Jenny J. who came to me for a face-lift. Her face was just fine, and I suggested instead a skin care regimen to alleviate fine lines. I didn't see Jenny again until a few months later, when I ran into her at a movie theater. She obviously had had the surgery elsewhere, and it was frustrating for me to realize that there is always a doctor somewhere who will do surgery, even on someone who doesn't truly benefit from it. In spite of the obvious changes to her face, this patient simply didn't look better. Jenny's eyes were unnaturally slanted, and her cheeks pulled in such a way that it would look artificial, even to a nonprofessional. On top of all that, she had two large scars on the sides of her face—definitely *not* the illusion of youth.

Always remember: Whether surgery is warranted or not, you ultimately will be able to find a surgeon who will tackle whatever is bothering you. Michael Jackson's face is caused by his surgeon. Jackson may be a patient who has body dysmorphism syndrome, which would mean he is never satisfied with his appearance. But it is the surgeon's responsibility to say no. Jackson's experience shows how consumer demand creates the market for a surgeon who will do almost anything.

The onset of middle age is a trying period for all of us. Marriages or careers are sometimes turned upside down, children leave home, our lifestyles change, the economy shifts, our friends move on, perhaps even depression sets in. At the same time, our physical energy fades, hormones fluctuate, hair turns gray, our bodies droop, and our skin turns thin and mottled. The combination of these events can result in a sense of desperation to stop the heady pace and reset the clock back a few years.

Patients in this age group need to understand that surgery does not alleviate wrinkles. Fine lines on the face are most often not caused by gravity but by motion (which surgeons call "animation") and by sun damage. They can most effectively be remedied with topical skin care, volumizing injections, or peeling techniques, not by surgery. Surgery only improves those signs of age that are caused by gravity: sagging jowls, large furrows, "turkey gobbler" chins, and droopy eyelids. Any facial surgery before these symptoms actually occur can be superfluous and can reshape one's face in an unnatural, "surgical" way. And now, for the first time, the current and imminent waves of bioengineered topical creams and other nonsurgical treatments offer noninvasive prevention or even *reversal* of fine lines on the face.

To me, personally, there is nothing worse than appearing "done," looking like you've had a face-lift. If someone else can tell you had a face-lift, then your surgeon has done you no service. Better to have nothing done at all than to appear "surgerized."

Many times, patients in this age group clamor for injections of collagen and other substances, as described in Chapter 6. I am not a great proponent of most unnatural filler injections. The effects are temporary—a few weeks, at most. Artecoll, Isolagen, Dermologen, Restylane, collagen, and the like are time-consuming and expensive investments, requiring you to return to the doctor again and again. In essence, the fact that there are so many different fillers indicates that they are not effective. All the new names and research mean manufacturers and doctors can charge you more money. (As I've mentioned before, the one exception to this rule is autologous fat transfer, which I highly recommend in most cases.)

Often, the frequent users of filler injections reach a point where they no longer receive any noticeable result—just as with a cream, overuse of filler injections can eventually neutralize their effects. These injections aren't harmful, as a rule. I just feel they are not effective in the long term. And there is nothing worse than the "First Wives Club" mannequin-like face of a woman who's had too many lip injections.

Botox is not a filler, and it can help prevent line formation by stopping the animation in parts of your face. Botox is physiologically different from filler injections, and I think in certain instances Botox injections are good, especially for those with deep furrows between the eyes. Botox can make these furrows disappear completely. One of my first patients told me that, after her Botox injection, people started to treat her better. When she had a scowl, they assumed she was not a pleasant woman.

Truly beautiful skin comes with a proper diet, exercise, a healthy spiritual condition, and a simple topical regimen that has no risks or side effects. This age range is a great time to perk up your exercise routine—even if you never really had one before—and to improve your diet. And this is the perfect time to begin a potent topical regimen, and perhaps "jump-start" it with a peel.

In addition to cleansing and moisturizing and avoiding the sun, the best skin therapy for this age group is using creams that reduce wrinkles. When I see someone in her late thirties, forties, or early fifties, I typically recommend a short-term combination regimen using Retin-A and a hydroquinone cream, along with RéVive. As I mentioned in Chapter 4, each of these creams affects the skin in different ways. Retin-A thickens the skin and increases its circulation, bleaching agents eliminate dark pigment spots by inhibiting the production of melanin, and RéVive increases the pace of new skin cell growth. As Retin-A works by inflaming the skin, I do recommend stopping this part of the regimen after three months. You do not need to use it constantly to see its effects, and it is good to take some time off from it. EGF and most bleaching agents are not inflammatory, and may be used year-round. After a year, you may resume using the Retin-A for another three months.

Naturally, these products must be used with sunscreen, as the sun's rays can reverse any benefits of these creams. In fact, I often tell a fair-skinned patient to use these topical products only during the winter months, because a lot of sun exacerbates redness. For those who think the colder seasons are too long and dark, I always tell my patients to look on the bright side: This time of year is wonderful for rejuvenating the complexion.

Sun damage is cumulative. Marti R., a forty-five-year-old actress, came to see me about the dozens of fine wrinkles and dark spots on her cheeks. She had not lain out in the sun since she was twenty-five, she told me. Even though she had avoided sun exposure for the last twenty years, those early days were still having their effects. Had she not lain out in the sun as a young woman—there is no question about it—her skin would have looked much smoother. Fortunately, a short dose of Retin-A, hydroquinone, and long-term use of RéVive can reverse much of the damage. After six months, Marti already looks fresh-faced and vibrant.

Because you are certain to get more sun exposure in the summer, no matter where you live and how hard you try to avoid it, I change this regimen for the summer months. The daily routine eliminates Retin-A during June, July, and August and replaces it with extra sunscreen, which is applied in the morning and then again at lunchtime. In September, you return Retin-A to the regimen, and continue with sunscreen applied just once a day.

AHAs are naturally occurring acids that stimulate skin turnover. The most commonly used AHA is glycolic acid, which derives from sugarcane. Others might include citric acid (from oranges and grapefruit), malic acid (from apples), and lactic acid (from milk). A good AHA cream contains at least 8 percent of the acid, with a low pH rating between 1 and 4. Anything with a pH between 5 and 7 won't have any noticeable effect on your skin except as a moisturizer.

MOST POPULAR NONSURGICAL COSMETIC PROCEDURES FOR PATIENTS AGED 51–64 PERFORMED IN 2003

Botox injection	799,038
Chemical peel	242,463
Collagen injection	218,639
Microdermabrasion	197,987
Sclerotherapy	144,135
Laser hair removal	92,234

A patient in her late thirties through early fifties benefits immensely from the effects of skin peels. The deeper peels (see Chapter 6) are the perfect treatment for someone at this age, and they are very safe. Nearly 99 percent of patients who have peels are very pleased with the outcome, and they tend to have realistic expectations. Start by having a superficial chemical peel (described on page 112), which requires several visits to a doctor. After one year, if you are not satisfied with the results, consider a laser peel, Obagi Blue Peel, or TCA peel. These can eliminate lip lines, age spots, rosacea, small moles, and acne scars.

Treat spider veins and excess facial hair with spot laser treatments, or RéVive Intensité Crème Lustre or Sans Veines Body Repair Cream, which contain IGF. The topical cream alone will reduce veins by 50 percent within five months. This cream rebuilds the inner matrix that supports the tiny blood vessels, so they become less dilated.

The VersaPulse laser emits a special light that seals shut spider veins, which are then reabsorbed into the body. The LightSheer Diode laser uses another shade of light that vaporizes the hair pigment and follicle. Lasers are superb for people who want to eliminate large freckles or deep age spots, tattoos, melasma from pregnancy, or rosacea, the middle-aged skin condition that commonly affects fair-skinned women. Lasers can target specific areas with deeper treatment and can be used on the face, hands, neck, or any area of the body.

If you are in your fifties, this is a good time to consider the more invasive phenol chemical peel or CO_2 laser peel, which can last for many years. But even a medium peel can be transforming when it is combined with Retin-A and hydroquinone.

EVERY DAY

Clean your face morning and night with a neutral product. Good facial cleansers include Cetaphil, Purpose, Neutrogena, and Basis. Just avoid any that contain alcohol, which is too drying.

Moisturize your face, neck, and hands after cleansing. Use products of your choosing from Oil of Olay, Neutrogena, Nivea, Lancôme, or Estée Lauder.

Every morning, apply sunscreen (minimum SPF 15) to your face, neck, and hands. During the summertime, reapply sunscreen at lunchtime. Your primary sun exposure comes not from going to the beach, but from simple daily errands out of doors. I do not think the higher Sun Protection Factor (SPF) numbers are as effective as simply applying any sunscreen twice a day instead of just once. There are many great brands in the stores, such as Shade, Almay, Lancôme, Neutrogena, and Coppertone, and also those from Avon Products. Make sure the sunscreen is effective against both UVA and UVB rays. The most effective sunscreens are those that physically block the sun, such as zinc oxide or micronized titanium oxide or the chemical block Parsol.

And of course, the best protection for your skin is to avoid the sun altogether. Even walking down the street on daily errands can cause sun damage to your skin. Wear a hat. Choose the shady sidewalk over the sunny side of the street. Sit at the table with the umbrella. If you are going to a sunny place or heading for the beach, use a sunblock, such as titanium oxide or zinc oxide cream.

Every evening, wash your face with a gentle makeup remover such as Almay or Lancôme. Moisturize.

Schedule a peel, or two—depending on the strength of your treatment. An annual peel of any kind will refresh your complexion and quickly erase the sun spots and fine lines that creep up from time to time. Mini-peels can even be done at a salon or spa.

Schedule a trip to a dermatologist, surgeon, or plastic surgeon. Each of these specialists is trained to identify and treat precancerous spots on your skin. Particularly during your forties and fifties, cumulative sun damage and genetics may cause the sudden appearance of basal cells or melanoma. The doctor should assess the skin all over your body for new or changing moles and freckles—they appear as frequently on the arms, legs, back, and chest as on the face.

Are Facials Helpful at All?

A facial can make you feel great—someone gently massaging your facial muscles while applying toners or masks. Extractions from your pores and mild exfoliation can brighten your complexion. But I'm not crazy about the prospect that bacteria may be lurking in such a busy setting. Choose your salon very carefully. If you get facials too frequently, they can start to become irritating, and even cause broken blood vessels. I also believe that many products used in salons are highly comedogenic, causing blocked pores and irritated skin. Go ahead and treat yourself once in a while, if these appeal to you, but I do not recommend more than one or two per year, at most.

It would be equally beneficial to your complexion if you opted instead for a full body massage. This gets your blood circulating, pumps oxygen into your muscles and tissues, and relaxes you even more than a facial does. Massages detoxify by increasing lymph flow into the body's waste bin; that is why frequently after a massage one has to urinate, even though there has been no increased hydration.

If you're pampering yourself at a salon, go for the massage instead of the facial from time to time. Your complexion will benefit, and so will the rest of you. Massage stimulates the flow of lymph, which is the clear liquid that you might see when you squeeze a pimple and the blood disappears. Lymph has its own circulatory system and is a mechanism for removal of waste and toxins from your skin.

Filler Injections

I consider collagen and other fillers overly expensive and time-consuming for such a short-term effect. But there is no doubt about the immediate results from such filler injections. I am most enthusiastic about the one injection that can last forever: fat injection.

A patient in her forties or fifties might well benefit from fat injections to alleviate undereye circles caused by troughs, frown lines, or vertical puppet lines along the chin. Except for silicone, the essence of all other fillers is the same, and they are temporary and expensive. As I described in Chapter 6, recent improvements in this procedure have made it more effective than ever. I see this procedure work very well on men, in particular. It is important to find a doctor who uses the new LipoStructure technique, however (see Resources, page 189). Fat injection does require extracting fat from another part of your body. Fine needles are used to draw out fat from your thighs, buttocks, or abdomen. For patients in this age group or older, fat injections are far and away a better option than other injections. When the new fat acquires a local blood supply, it can become a permanent filler. I hope to see this underrated procedure outpace other fillers in the years to come.

When you receive an injection, most doctors "overfill" the

area, to allow for some immediate reabsorption. The swelling abates after a couple of days. Whichever injection you choose, you should be aware that they might all be temporary. The duration of injections relies on a person's individual body receptiveness, skin quality, and lifestyle. What works for your friend may not work so well for you. Your doctor will evaluate your facial components and help you arrive at the treatment that works best for you.

Undereye circles occur from different causes. In dark- or olive-skinned patients, undereye circles are often caused by natural pigmentation. Surgery has no effect on this condition—only bleaching creams can diminish this undereye discoloration. In other cases, undereye circles are caused by the pooling of blood within the "fat pads" of the lower lids. This is particularly true for fair skin types. Allergies can accentuate the pooling. Since the skin is so thin in this region, the pooled blood shows through the skin as a dark circle. These circles can be remedied by simply removing the fat in a classic lower eyelid lift (blepharoplasty) or by using RéVive Intensité Les Yeux with IGF and MPI. These bioengineered ingredients restructure the blood vessels so they are not as dilated.

A third cause of undereye circles is the trough that may start to appear while you're in your mid-thirties. The trough appears because of the loss of volume that naturally occurs with aging. The actual trough is due to the orbital rim—the bone—showing through the skin. It can be treated in several ways. One is a special type of blepharoplasty that is often part of a mid-face lift. The bags are not removed but rather repositioned to eliminate the trough. Another procedure is fat injection around the bags and orbital rim, restoring lost volume to eliminate the trough. These are definitive but rather invasive treatments. Using the topical cream RéVive Intensité Les Yeux will naturally stimulate some of the volume to return, often in just eight weeks.

INJECTABLES AT A GLANCE

Name	Description	Purpose	Risks	Results
Zyderm/ Zyplast	Collagen injections made from purified cow skin	Fills wrinkles, scars on face, around lips	Allergic reaction	Immediate; lasts up to 6 months
Cymetra (micronized Alloderm)	Human tissue collagen matrix derived from cadaver tissue	Filler for lips, nasolabial folds, deep wrinkles	Bruising	Multiple treatments needed; lasts 2 months
CosmoDerm/ CosmoPlast	Derived from human tissue that has been grown in a laboratory	Fills frown lines, crow's-feet, forehead lines, lip lines, marionette lines	Bruising	Immediate; lasts up to 6 months
Fascian	Injectable made from tissue of patient's thigh muscle	Stimulates collagen; adds bulk	Bruising	Lasts up to 6 months
Autologen/ Dermalogen	Derived from patient's skin and processed for injection	Alternative to traditional collagen	Bruising; expensive	2 or 3 treatments; not permanent
Plasmagel	Plasma emulsion derived from patient's blood and vitamin C complex	Soft tissue filler to add volume	Bruising	Lasts up to 3 months

Name	Description	Purpose	Risks	Results
Fat	Injections using fat from patient's abdomen, buttocks, or thigh	Adds volume; fills wrinkles, enhances lips	bruising	Usually permanent
Botox	Botulinum toxin type A	Smooths wrinkles; fills forehead lines	Bruising; numbness, droopy eyelids; immunity possible with long-term use	Effective in 2 weeks; lasts up to 6 months
Mybloc	Botulinum toxin type B	Smooths wrinkles	Bruising, numbness, droopy eyelids, possible immunity	Faster-acting than Botox; lasts up to 6 months
Dysport	Botulinum toxin type A	Smooths wrinkles	Same as above; not yet approved by FDA in U.S.	Claims to last twice as long as Botox
Restylane/ Perlane	Synthetic hyaluronic acid	Soft tissue filler; adds volume	Redness, swelling	Immediate; lasts up to 1 year

Name	Description	Purpose	Risks	Results
Hylaform/ Juvederm	Hyaluronic acid derived from rooster combs	Soft tissue filler; adds volume	Redness, swelling; allergy	Lasts up to 6 months
Artecoll	75% bovine collagen and 25% polymethyl-methacrylate polymers as "micro implant"	Permanent filler that encourages collagen production	Clumping; rash	Immediate; maximum use every 3 months
Radiance (Bioform)	Calcium hydroxylapatite, a natural substance found in bones and teeth, made into injectable paste	Adds volume; encourages collagen formation	Clumping	Immediate; lasts up to 5 years

DR. BROWN'S NONSURGICAL OPTIONS FOR PATIENTS 36–55

Forehead creases	Botox
	Laser resurfacing
	Retin-A, intermittently
	RéVive EGF or Intensité Cream
Crow's-feet	Retin-A
	Chemical or laser peel
	Botox
Lip lines	Fat injection
	Laser peel

	Chemical peel
	Dermabrasion
	RéVive Lip Cream
Sagging jowls	Fat injection
	CO_2 laser peel
	Thermage
Nasolabial fold	Fat injection
	Filler injection
	RéVive Intensité Cream
Marionette lines	Fat injection
	RéVive Intensité Cream
Droopy neck	Liposuction
	Fat injection
	Thermage
Spider veins	Laser therapy
	RéVive Sans Veines Body Repair Cream
	RéVive Intensité Crème Lustre
	Sclerotherapy
Undereye circles	RéVive Intensité Les Yeux
	Autologous fat injections

The Role of Aging Hormones

In the preceding chapter, I discussed the effects on a woman's complexion of birth control medications. The changes in aging skin are subsequently affected by menopause and hormone replacement therapy (HRT). Estrogen, testosterone, the body's natural steroid dyhydroepiandrosterone (DHEA), melatonin, and human growth hormone (HGH) all decline with age. Many are now aware of the risks to the cardiovascular system when they use hormone supplements, as revealed by the National Institute of Aging and the Women's Health Initiative in their long-term clinical trials, which concluded that the risks to women's health outweighed the benefits.

Aging decreases one's natural production of growth hormone and, subsequently, the human production of IGF. Some people experience huge decreases in the growth hormone—it varies with your genetic history. This loss has its greatest effects on the cognitive functions of the brain, but it also shows on the face with the loss of IGF protein, which results in decreasing tissues under the skin. Hormone replacement therapy helps maintain healthy levels of protein and volume in your skin. But many women cannot or choose not to use HRT for a variety of other health reasons. The benefits of HRT have not been proven to outweigh the health risks, and it is not an issue that should be determined by one's desire for younger skin. To that end, however, the IGF protein has been bioengineered for risk-free use in a topical cream, available as Intensité Cream from Ré-Vive. Tests showed that after using IGF for five months, the skin's matrix—its "glue"—is noticeably improved and the skin retained more overall succulent fluid content. This means your skin can benefit from a topical replacement therapy that does not affect the rest of your body. Intensité helps add lost volume to your face.

Only 35 percent of all adults over the age of sixty-five have "normal" levels of human growth hormone. Most of us have lower and lower levels as we get older, which causes volume loss in our tissues, muscles, and bones. Clinics have sprouted up across the country, promising a virtual fountain of youth through injections of human growth hormone. But no one yet knows the long-term effects of growth hormone replacement therapy on healthy aging adults. Until more studies have been completed, I do not recommend this treatment just to achieve youthful skin, particularly when there are so many safe and effective alternatives.

Action Plan: Nonsurgical Options for Ages 36–55

This list shows optimal procedures available now, and also some of the options that will be available to you in the immediate future.

THIS YEAR

- laser or chemical peel
- fat injection
- RéVive Cream with EGF
- RéVive Intensité with IGF, KGF, and MPI

IN ONE YEAR

- Pulse light or photodynamic laser peel

IN TWO YEARS

- Actizyme cream for power exfoliation

IN FIVE TO TEN YEARS

- Scarless face-lift
- Innovative hormone replacement therapy
- Deep RF or LED peel
- Telomerase creams for genetic repair of the skin

When Surgery Might Work Best

Very often, those who undergo the knife at this age to make themselves appear younger are disappointed—either by the startling changes in their appearance, or by not feeling changed "enough." The exception for this age group would be someone who has lost a lot of weight, shows excessive results of gravity or sun damage, or has loose skin around the neck.

Most face-lifts involve two things: removing excess facial skin and tightening the tissues (muscles, fat, and fascia) beneath the skin. The tissue under the facial skin is called subcutaneous musculoapomneurotic substance (SMAS) and is a thin, fibrous tissue. We tighten the layers and drape the skin over the tightened tissue, using a scalpel or a laser. There are newer face-lift techniques that go deeper than this (such as a subperiosteal mid-face face-lift, where the tissues are actually separated from the facial bones and then lifted).

Losing weight is often the cure for double chins, and some turkey gobbler necks, much as some patients prefer not to hear this. Mary K., a fifty-four-year-old attorney, came to see me about a face-lift. She was an ample woman with a petite frame and blond hair, whose skin was freckled and papery. She was bothered by her double chin but, as I pointed out to her, most of it was fat. Mary was fifteen pounds overweight. I gave her my list of optimal foods with which to prepare her own diet, as well as my topical regimen. She returned in three months, looking fantastic and ten pounds thinner. There was no surgical procedure I could have performed to transform her face so magnificently.

Sometimes, people in this age group are concerned about furrowed foreheads, which can make you look tired. For these patients, I might recommend an endoscopic brow lift, which is described in Chapter 12. This is not to be confused with a "mini face-lift." I do not think there is anything "mini" about having surgery. If you are going to the expense and trouble of having a surgical procedure, it should be because you have an abnormal amount of excess skin. An endoscopic brow lift can open up eyes by raising the brows. Under sedation, three one-inch incisions are made behind the hairline. A lighted scope is inserted, allowing the surgeon to work under the skin to lift the brow tissue and secure it in a higher position. It is an almost imperceptible change that transforms the eyes. This is a wonderful operation because it is never obvious (unless it is overdone, of course). It makes women so pretty, enhancing the distance between the lash lines and the eyebrow. It may make you feel as stunning as a movie star. Lines and wrinkles, of course, are still best treated with creams and peels.

One of the most common and least noticeable surgical procedures is eyelid surgery, or blepharoplasty. This is where excess skin and fat are removed from the area between the eye and the eyebrow. It doesn't change the shape or placement of the eyebrow, but opens up eyes that have heavy or puffy lids. Not only are the upper or "hooded" eyelids reparable, but so are the lower eyelids. Bags can be removed or repositioned, and the incision can be on the inside of the eyelid so it is truly scarless. This is a simple procedure with a very high rate of patient satisfaction.

MOST POPULAR SURGICAL PROCEDURES FOR WOMEN AGED 51–64 PERFORMED IN 2003

Eyelid surgery	108,880
Face-lift	76,565
Liposuction	56,203
Nose reshaping	44,768
Brow lift	28,325
Tummy tuck	20,273

In my experience, one of the greater risks of surgery that is virtually untreatable is the patient's disappointment with the outcome. No matter how many pre-op and post-op photos and computer graphics are shown, and how many conversations with doctors are held about the realities of the outcomes, this is a real pitfall of surgery. Patricia A. was a forty-eight-year-old housewife who came to me for a brow lift and blepharoplasty. Everything went smoothly and her eyes became free of bags and puffiness but, after she recovered fully, she felt she did not look different enough. She agreed that the surgery accomplished what she'd requested, but she had a lingering sense of disappointment. Her expectations had been that her whole face would be turned back to twenty. If you are determined to pursue surgical procedures during this part of your life, Chapter 12 explains and illustrates the optimal procedures.

Interestingly, I find that simpler peels and topical treatments have not only a physical effect, but an emotional one as well. Some women feel very guilty about the prospect of cosmetic enhancement, particularly about having surgery. I don't know whether they feel overly self-indulgent or vain, but a lot of women feel that it is "bad" to have cosmetic surgery—the cost is enormous, there are risks, and it causes pain. As a plastic surgeon, I know cosmetic surgery is wonderful and safe, but it is never necessary. By using non-invasive procedures and bioengineered creams, many women not only see their wrinkles disappear, but no longer feel the lingering guilt associated with having cosmetic surgery.

Some people say that, by your fifties, you have the face you deserve. But I believe that you have the face you deserve after you've erased your wrinkles. A topical regimen is often more satisfying to someone seeking rejuvenation.

Get Moving

Healthy skin requires a lot of oxygen—from the outside and from the inside. That's why you hear so many doctors recommend drinking a lot of water, and I do too. Another way to inject your bloodstream with increased oxygen is by breathing more, and one way to do that is to get a little exercise.

I started doing yoga when I was in my forties, and I was not in the best physical condition. I noticed immediate improvement in my skin tone and my energy levels. T'ai chi is another practice that is gentle on the joints and well suited for the onset of middle age. Pilates exercises also strengthen your muscular core by simplifying and conditioning your body's exertion. Pilates can significantly increase mobility. Yoga and t'ai chi classes are now available in cities across the country. These practices are perfect for people with bad joints, and for those who are just starting on an exercise regimen after years of going without.

I recommend going to a yoga or t'ai chi class twice a week. In addition, I recommend going for a brisk walk or climbing stairs twice a week as well. Treadmills and other exercise machines are very effective (and they keep you out of the sun!). Swimming is great for toning your body and restoring oxygen, but you must be careful to use sunscreen, then clean and moisturize your skin afterward.

Women who are currently in their sixties and seventies did not have the topical skin care options in their forties that you have now. There is a wide array of accessible, safe, noninvasive treatments that will bring immediate improvements to your appearance. In addition, these products will slow down the aging process of your skin over the long term. By the time you are in your sixties and seventies, you will look younger than those who are that age now. You may be middle-aged, but we live at a time that has redefined the "prime" of our lives. You are just at the beginning. If you are in your forties or fifties, don't miss the opportunity to extend your prime years of beauty.

CHAPTER 10

over 55: immediate and
long-lasting rejuvenation

S ome may object to my writing a chapter that combines treatment for a fifty-six-year-old with that for an eighty-year-old. This age group spans an entire generation, and I don't mean to imply that anyone approaching sixty looks the same as someone in her eighties. The common denominator for this group is that all patients have skin with similar qualities and needs. As with every age group, the severity of facial lines and wrinkles may be vastly different from one individual to another. For example, Mary C. is in her late eighties, but she looks twenty years younger than that. She has a few wrinkles around her eyes, but her complexion still shines because she has no age spots or excessive facial hair. Another patient of mine, Carl B., is only sixty-two and looks eighty. He has never used sunscreen and has a dozen very dark pigment spots on his face that will probably, one by one, develop basal cell symptoms. He has deep nasolabial folds and his earlobes are very large. Even though Carl and Mary have skin that has aged very differently, the preferred treatment options are similar, regardless of specific age. There are a number of elements that affect your facial appearance at this age—sun damage, dynamic wrinkles, gravity, bone and tissue loss, hormone decline, and, well, hair.

Thin Out the Peach Fuzz

In the years after menopause, women's low estrogen levels prompt the loss of bone structure, muscle, tissue, and skin thickness. Both men and women also suffer from thinning hair as our metabolism slows down. For women, this is compounded by the development of excessive facial hair. Diminishing this downy facial hair is a good first step in rejuvenating your look. You may not be all that aware of your increased facial hair—it is colorless, and it may never have been a problem for you before. But this fine facial hair grows longer and thicker after menopause, and it clouds the brightness and smoothness of your complexion. For some patients, facial hair is still negligible at this age. Assessing this condition and treating it, if necessary, is a helpful first step toward cosmetic rejuvenation.

Most women find electrolysis very painful, and rightly so. Having an electrode squeezed into your hair follicle for a jolt of electricity sounds like a barbaric treatment today. And an hour-long session of painful electrolysis results in the removal of about forty hairs. Not long ago, lasers started to be used for painless hair removal, but it only worked if the hair had darker color. Most facial hair does not contain any pigment, so lasers were not often used. But newer lasers can zap all facial hair, no matter what color it is. I highly recommend to most women over the age of sixty that they have a professional laser treatment to reduce their facial hair. It is not expensive, and only requires a few treatments to achieve permanent hair reduction.

Of course, you may also try over-the-counter creams designed for temporary facial depilation. Some of these are very irritating, however. Test a sample on your forearm before putting it on your face.

Daily Regimen

Wash your face and neck with gentle cleansers such as Cetaphil, Oil of Olay, or fragrance-free Dove. Thank heavens, you are finally at an age where acne is no longer a problem! Moisturize with a day cream that contains sunscreen, such as Eucerin Extra Protective Moisturizing Lotion SPF 30, Neutrogena Healthy Defense Daily Moisturizer SPF 30, Olay Complete Total Effects or Age-Defying Protective Renewal Lotion SPF 15. At night, use a heavier moisturizer, and don't forget to apply it to your neck, hands, and forearms. Good brands include Neutrogena, Estée Lauder, Prescriptives, RéVive, and Oil of Olay.

Use AHA moisturizers on the rest of your body. You might also use it on your face in a combination regimen with Retin-A, which will show remarkable improvement.

Bioengineered Creams Work Even Better at This Age

Contrary to what some people believe, patients over fifty-five benefit more than others from bioengineered topical treatment. The visible results from creams containing EGF, KGF, MPI, or IGF are astonishing. The effects are much more remarkable than those from nontechnical botanical creams such as Kinerase or StriVectin SD, the stretch-mark cream that many people now use on their faces. The changes are even more remarkable when accompanied by a lower-calorie, sugar-free diet and even a minimal amount of exercise. No other age group shows such immediate and dramatic results. In only a couple of weeks, these patients have fewer wrinkles, smoother skin, and a brighter overall tone.

My seventy-nine-year-old friend Connie has spent a lot of time in the sun. She loves to work in the garden and play golf. She learned to use sunscreen later in life, and now wears a hat when she's outdoors. But her face is still smooth and clear. She started using EGF cream back when she was in her early sixties, when I was performing the first tests on it. Her complexion has hardly aged since then. When you slow down the aging process with a topical cream such as EGF, the effect accumulates. After nearly twenty years of using EGF, someone who is nearly eighty will look twenty years younger, like Connie.

When I first met Anna L., she was seventy-five years old and had never had any special treatment on her face. She was active and healthy, but she felt her face looked baggy and dull. We gave her a medium peel, and she started using RéVive as well as Retin-A. The results of these treatments were virtually immediate: Her skin lost its mottled spots and acquired a porcelain tone. But we noticed her hands looked older than her face. Anna had veiny "grandma" hands. People underestimate or ignore the appearance of their hands. But it is essential to treat them if you want to look and feel completely rejuvenated.

Your Hands Speak Volumes

We smoothed out Anna's hands with fat injections, so they became less bony and veiny. Anna also applied the RéVive and

Retin-A creams to her hands, and added her sunblock routine to them as well. If you are over sixty, your hands may have thin, dry skin, pigment spots, blotches, veins, and bony joints. Here are several options for improving the appearance of your hands:

- Topical creams such as Retin-A, bleaching agents, or RéVive can help exfoliate and even out dark spots.

- Microdermabrasion works as well on hands as it does on the face, polishing your hands and reducing sun damage.

- Chemical peels can work very well to rejuvenate the skin on your hands.

- Intense Pulsed Light can reduce the signs of aging as well as stimulate collagen production for thicker skin.

- Fat injections can restore the soft tissue and fill out furrows between your finger bones.

- Sclerotherapy is an injection of saline solution into the veins, which then causes veins to disappear.

- New creams containing MDI Complex, such as Skin Therapy Advanced B5 Serum or RéVive Sans Veines Body Cream with MPI, reproduce the healthy balance of human enzymes and their inhibitors. These creams strengthen the protective function of the skin and eliminate redness, lines, age spots, and spider veins.

My general recommendation to any patient in this age group is to treat the back of your hands with the same elements that you use on your face. Your hands are an important part of your appearance and need to be treated with the same delicate care.

The effects of chemical and laser peels on patients aged fifty-five and over are incredible. I wouldn't hesitate to recommend that every patient over sixty try a medium chemical peel. There are no open wounds or scars, and you can resume normal activity in a week. But be sure you precede the peel with six weeks of topical creams such as Retin-A, hydroquinone, and RéVive. These creams actually allow the peel to penetrate more deeply, and they help to speed healing. You can get a medium peel every two years and have a glow for the rest of your life. Microdermabrasion is another good option for a patient over sixty.

Erbium laser peels can have even greater effects than a medium peel on patients of this age. If you have severe "cobweb" wrinkles all over your face, you might consider a CO_2 laser peel, which is much stronger than the erbium laser. A CO_2 laser uses carbon dioxide to create the laser beam, and its effects are as powerful and enduring as a phenol peel. The CO_2 laser actually shrinks skin and gives the face a different sort of lift.

Injections

Filler injections have become enormously popular with patients in their forties and fifties, but I don't see them as an important element for improving the appearance of someone over sixty. Why not? Well, this patient is more likely to have wrinkled skin and sagging from gravity, neither of which are really helped by injections. I think it would be a waste to spot-treat crow's-feet, lip creases, or frown lines, when the whole face would improve tremendously from a peel. The peel would not only reduce lines targeted by fillers, but it would refresh the overall tone, and last much longer.

The effects can be maintained with topical skin creams. I do not recommend that women over sixty waste their time and money with repeated filler injections such as collagen, or even Botox. Invest instead in a larger treatment such as a peel, which will have longer-lasting effects. Many doctors don't agree with me, as attested by the large numbers of patients who still seek out filler injections. But injections simply aren't appropriate or practical remedies for patients over sixty.

MOST POPULAR NONSURGICAL TREATMENTS FOR THOSE OVER AGE 65 PERFORMED IN 2003

Laser hair removal	81,280
Microdermabrasion	66,491
Botox injection	60,182
Laser peel	44,384
Chemical peel	18,966
Collagen injection	18,866

Hormone Therapy

As we age, the loss of bone and muscle mass affects the shapes of our faces. The chin recedes, the nose droops, the jawline fades. There are currently several clinical studies in progress involving the use of human growth hormone and resistance training to offset these deficiencies, which have had astounding results. As I mentioned earlier, the "off-label" use of growth hormone injections as an antiaging treatment has become more common, and there are even over-the-counter products such as mouth sprays that contain recombinant HGH. But its long-term risks are not yet known. Short-term risks include carpal tunnel syndrome, blood sugar problems, aching joints, acne, and weight gain. I do not recommend systemic use of HGH as an antiaging therapy.

Topical creams containing estrogen have long been marketed for vaginal irritation. Premarin cream, for example, stimulates collagen and rebuilds thicker skin. I have seen studies where doctors prescribe Premarin for use on facial skin, and it appears to have similar effects. After a month, the face is smoother, with fewer lines and wrinkles. The long-term effects are not known, but estrogen cream has been shown to be quite safe. The same is true for progesterone creams. They may not really have any effect on your facial skin, but they are not overly harmful. I would not use any of these for more than four months per year, however.

One-third of all adults in their senior years maintain normal, healthy levels of growth hormone. Muscle mass and bone density can be much more safely maintained by following a modest exercise routine.

Exercise

The good news for people in this age group is this: It does not require an enormous amount of exertion for you to provide your skin with revitalizing oxygen. If you go for a brisk walk three times a week, for forty-five minutes each time, you will provide your entire body with enormous benefits. The bad news: If you do not do at least a little walking or weight-bearing exercise (meaning that you are on your feet, carrying your own weight), your muscles and bones will waste away. This is true for the bones and muscles in the face, as well as for the rest of your body.

It is also amazingly effective to do a little weight/resistance training, such as lifting two-pound hand weights over your head.

Repeating this twelve times, three days a week, can build up your bone mass and increase circulation throughout your body.

If you are prevented from moving because of joint injury or arthritis, take a pain reliever and exercise anyway. Take as much pain reliever (or glucosamine) as you can to keep yourself moving, as long as you are then moving normally and not limping or causing further injury. The best exercise routine for patients over sixty is walking back and forth in a waist-high pool of water for thirty minutes, two or three times a week. This exercise will actually help decrease your pain over the long term, and it will remove stress lines from your face.

Get Your Legs Working

More than half of all adults over the age of sixty suffer from varicose veins. These are veins whose valves have stopped working properly, so the blood flows irregularly. This causes the veins to become thick and bulging. As a result, many people suffer from leg pain, night cramps, and fatigue. These symptoms sometimes lead to eczema, hemorrhage, ulcers, swelling, or blood clots. As a result, these patients may unknowingly avoid any activity that requires them to stand. Walking is still a great benefit for these patients, however. Varicose veins are now easily cured, and it's worth doing if you want to maintain health and vitality for as many years as possible.

Many people don't feel pain but simply don't like the way their veins look. There are now a number of noninvasive, nonsurgical procedures to eliminate varicose veins.

One of them is laser treatment, which has a 98 percent success rate with very low recurrence (much better results than the old surgical removal method). The EndoVenous Laser Treatment (EVLT) uses heat from a laser to close the saphenous vein, the large blood vessel in the thigh that is the source of most varicose veins. Using ultrasound for direction, the small laser fiber is inserted into the vein and pulses of light are emitted. EVLT can be done in an hour with a local anesthetic, leaves no scars, and recovery is almost immediate. It costs about $3,000 per leg (much less than surgery) and is available across the country. A similar treatment uses a radio frequency instead of laser.

Another option is sclerotherapy, which is a simple injection of fluid into the veins that causes them to disintegrate.

Don't forget to be equally attentive to your feet. If they cause you problems or prevent you from walking, consult a podiatrist and seek out proper walking shoes. It doesn't make sense to let your whole body weaken and age faster simply because you have a painful toe.

Lifestyle

Once you pass sixty, you do not need a calorie intake as high as you once needed for energy. Your calorie intake should be not much more than 1,000 per day for women, and 2,000 per day for men. It matters how you get these calories too: Green vegetables, fish, meat, and milk products become more vital to your health at this age. I do think calcium supplements are important for this age group, as they have been proven to prevent bone loss from your facial structure.

It is also now common knowledge that social activity and mental stimulation can prevent cardiovascular disease, diabetes, even cancer. Activities such as working, playing bridge, gardening, or playing music are better for your body than sitting, watching TV, and overeating. Be vigilant about stimulating your body and your mind, and your skin will continue to be stimulated as well.

If a woman is going to have surgery, her late fifties can be a great age for a face-lift, as this age most often starts to show the effects of gravity around the eyes and chin. This depends on a woman's inherent aging process, of course. Although I believe the skin creams alleviate wrinkles and help all patients to look younger, this is an age group that can benefit from aesthetic surgery more than any other. After all, someone in her sixties is less likely than a twenty-year-old to benefit from the innovations not yet on the market. And the earlier you have surgery, the longer its effects will last.

Along with the mouth, our eyebrows indicate most of our emotions. Eyebrow position can make us look happy, tired, angry, or sad. The eyebrow position tells others in an instant what our emotional status is. Low, flat eyebrows indicate fatigue. Eyebrows that point up to the middle look sad. Downward slanting eyebrows look angry, while high arches look happy.

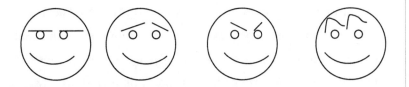

Over time, gravity causes our eyebrows to sag. Our eyelids appear heavier, making a person look tired all the time. Many of us don't even realize it, but we frequently raise our eyebrows to lift the lid off our eyes. This causes forehead lines, of course. Sometimes this can be temporarily corrected with Botox injections, but the best treatment is to have brow-lift surgery. This is now performed with an endoscopic camera, which allows the surgeon to see beneath the skin without having to make large incisions. Recovery takes just a few days—much quicker than recovery from traditional surgery.

Endoscopic surgery is relatively noninvasive. It has been used for years for knee surgery and tubal ligations and, in recent years, has become a superb tool for facial surgery. The endoscope itself is merely a viewing device—small incisions must still be made behind the hairline for small surgical instruments. Endoscopy can also be used for a moderate tummy tuck, breast augmentation, forehead lift, and face-lifts. Many patients who have a brow lift also have eyelid surgery at the same time. This removes excess skin and fat just beneath the brow.

In my opinion, the brow lift is the least invasive surgical procedure that provides the most noticeable improvements. It can simply open up a woman's face to a new radiance. I've focused this section on aesthetic surgery for female patients, who receive 80 percent of such procedures in this country. Men are more of a challenge. At this age, they may notice extended earlobes or a longer nose. These can be remedied with very simple surgical procedures, and may be all a man needs to regain a youthful look. But men who have too many other surgical procedures can start to look very feminine—witness some older movie stars and male celebrities whose eyebrows look out of place and they appear to be elderly women. A respectable surgeon will work sparingly on a man to prevent this.

If you have a "turkey gobbler" chin or heavy jowls, you should consider some of the more advanced treatments, described in Chapter 12. But once again, surgery cannot re-create youth. A face-lift does not improve the quality of your skin or restore the volume of youth. This can only be done on the molecular level. The new topical creams and peels do this—in fact, they provide much more rejuvenation at this age than at any other.

MOST POPULAR SURGICAL PROCEDURES FOR THOSE OVER 65 PERFORMED IN 2003

Eyelid surgery	37,107
Face-lift	22,774
Nose reshaping	10,554
Brow lift	8,233
Liposuction	7,170

CHAPTER 11

no matter what your age, change with the seasons

ust as the weather changes from winter to spring and summer to autumn, so should your skin care regimen change with the seasons. As the largest influence on the condition of your skin, the sun should be your signal to rotate how you are taking care of your largest organ. Each of you has a different routine, and different needs for proper skin care, so what you do will vary from what your friends might do. But not enough patients pay attention to the effects of the sun throughout the year.

Here are some basic rules to follow, when adjusting for weather and changes in the power of the sun.

Winter

- Increase your daily use of moisturizer, or choose a richer, heavier cream.

- Apply moisturizer not only on your face but all over your body. Do it at least twice a day, if it feels good!

- Oily skin still needs to be moisturized! Use an oil-free or less oily product.

- Use alpha hydroxy or glycolic acid products, or Retin-A, to keep your skin exfoliated. Use less frequently if your skin becomes too dry.

- Get a fruit acid peel at a salon every other month.

- Apply sunscreen (SPF 15) to your face every morning.

- If you take a winter vacation somewhere warm, get a self-tanning treatment before you go, so you won't be tempted to bask out in the sun. I don't mean a tanning booth—stay away from artificial light rays just as you would the sun itself. But the new applications of self-tanning lotions are wonderful, either as a "buff 'n' bronze" massage in a salon, in a "spray booth," or in the form of over-the-counter creams available in drugstores. It is important to exfoliate your body before applying these yourself—and be sure to wash your hands well after application.

  While in the sun, stay under a wide-brimmed hat and wear more sunscreen—SPF 30. As good as the hot sun may feel right now, it is performing extra damage to your pale skin.

- Since you're indoors most of the time, winter is a good time to have a deeper peel, such as a medium chemical peel or laser peel. By the time spring arrives, you will be fully recovered and ready to show off your new glowing complexion.

- Your pale skin may also reveal age spots or little red veins on your face—consult a doctor about spot treatment with lasers.

- Pay more attention to using hand creams—your hands are

feeling the weather as much as your face. Winter skin is much more easily traumatized.

- Manicures can help control hangnails and dry nails of winter.
- Shed those holiday pounds by resuming a stricter eating pattern.
- Enroll in a dance or yoga class.
- Perform your own "ABCD" skin checks for unusual moles or deepening freckles.

Spring

- Greater humidity may bring on some acne—change to a light or oil-free facial moisturizer.
- Schedule an appointment with your dermatologist for your annual skin cancer checkup. May is Skin Cancer Awareness Month!
- Start applying sunscreen not only in the morning but again at midday.
- Make sure your children also wear sunscreen, particularly on the face.
- Shop for hats and visors—straw hats do not prevent UVA rays from hitting your face.
- Do some spring cleaning of your skin products, including makeup. Anything more than one year old is not something you want to put on your skin!
- Start using bronzer makeup, but use lighter-weight foundations. The oilier products of winter should be phased out of your makeup application.

- Consult a doctor about laser removal of excess hair.

- Buy new sunscreens—the jars from last year are no longer effective. Sunscreens and self-tanners have quite a short shelf life—no more than three months.

- Apply sunscreen thirty minutes before going outside in the morning, and then again at lunchtime.

- You can cut back on your use of moisturizers—let the humidity in the fresh air do it for you!

- Take a break from Retin-A, although other creams are fine to use in summer. Stop using Retin-A from May through October. Your skin will remain clear if you add more sunscreen instead.

- If you have oily skin, you may need to treat yourself with Oxy 10 or Clearasil during the humid summer months, to keep blemishes away. These contain benzoyl peroxide.

- Get regular light fruit acid peels to refresh your complexion through the warmer months.

- Wear a hat—every day. Some people do not like how they look in hats, but the difference in your skin's condition will more than make up for this inconvenience.

- Protect your eyes (and prevent crow's-feet) by wearing sunglasses when you are outdoors. Hats and sunglasses are particularly important if you start exercising more out in the fresh air. You must wear these, even when jogging, biking, or playing tennis.

- When sitting or lying outdoors, or swimming, cover your entire face with clear zinc oxide. Reapply frequently.

- Use self-tanning lotions or sprays for a bronze glow.

- Your skin contains much more moisture in the summer months, and may be able to tolerate creams and products that were too harsh for your skin in the wintertime. This is a good time to experiment with new skin products.

Fall

- Resume your nightly regimen with Retin-A, in addition to your other face creams. But remember to stop after three months.

- Continue to apply sunscreen every morning.

- Consult a doctor about getting your spider veins and varicose veins treated, either with sclerotherapy, laser treatment, or Ré-Vive Sans Veines cream.

- Consider the options for getting a laser peel or chemical peel. This can be done before the holidays and you can enjoy the immediate results while the sun is less powerful.

- Visit a spa and treat yourself to a massage, a facial, a pedicure, and a makeup consultation.

- Start applying moisturizer all over your body, as much as two times a day.

- Start using a lip cream to keep away chapped lips. Reapply it frequently during colder months. Try to avoid lip balm that contains camphor or eucalyptus, which can cause inflammation and addictive usage. (Lip balms with camphor actually make your lips more chapped.)

- Change your makeup to accommodate your paler skin—get a makeover in a department store.

- Install a humidifier in your bedroom and/or office. This makes a great difference in the condition of your skin.

- Switch to a creamier cleanser for your face and body. Stop using face products that contain alcohol.

- Work out at a health club and go to the steam room. This is great for the skin, the circulation, and feels great in the colder months.

CHAPTER 12

other advanced procedures

This book is dedicated to attaining younger skin without surgery, but there are selected aging conditions that cannot otherwise be corrected. In the twentieth century, the desire to alter your appearance with surgery was seen as a weakness, a by-product of an "inferiority complex." Today, such a desire is a sign of strength, a pragmatic, healthy response to the demands of our modern world. What was known as an "inferiority complex" is now called "self-esteem." The most common aesthetic surgical procedures today are breast enhancement and liposuction. They are in great demand by women of all ages and incomes.

I do not recommend facial procedures without serious consideration of their risks and benefits. A patient must feel there is no alternative, even after reading this book. This chapter includes guidelines for determining which advanced procedure might be right for you, as well as specific risks and side effects, and the overall life span of their results.

Recently, the Mayo Clinic performed a study on women who had face-lifts in the early 1970s. The average age at surgery was about sixty-one years old. Their study revealed that these women lived as much as ten years longer than their peers who did not have a face-lift. These patients, who were all women, seemed to have a greater commitment to maintaining overall health and fitness. Researchers attribute their longevity to enhanced self-esteem and a brighter outlook on life. I think this now applies to patients who use less invasive procedures, such as peels and topical creams. However, you should be informed about what is involved with advanced procedures.

Here is an overview of most aesthetic surgery options. You should consult a plastic surgeon to help determine if one of these procedures is appropriate for you. Make sure he or she is board-certified by the American Board of Plastic Surgery (ABPS), and not by a board with a different name. Dermatologists may perform certain other procedures, but they are not surgeons and most do not have admission privileges at hospitals. If anything should go wrong—a rare occurrence, but be realistic—your physician might need to transfer you immediately to a hospital; however, most dermatologists would not have the credentials to do so.

Abdominoplasty (tummy tuck)

This surgery flattens the abdomen by removing excess fat and tightening the muscles with sutures in the abdominal wall. The surgery takes up to four hours, under general sedation, and recovery can take up to four weeks. There is a wide scar across the lower abdomen (under the bikini line), which fades after several months. This procedure is often chosen by women who have been pregnant, and who want to tighten the skin and eliminate stretch marks. This is a major surgical procedure, and is not as simple as a "tuck." Some patients have this done if they require a hysterectomy. It can also serve to strengthen the lower spine, as tightening the abdominal wall provides greater support to the lumbar area. The average surgeon's fee for this procedure in 2002 was $4,739.

Breast Enlargement

This surgical procedure increases the size of breasts by using implants filled with saline. It takes less than two hours to perform, and the patient is usually up and around within a couple of days. There are some risks of bleeding, infection, scar tissue, and moving of the implants. The results are permanent. Average 2002 surgeon's fee: $3,436.

Breast Lift

This surgery raises and reshapes sagging breasts by removing excess skin and repositioning the nipple. This procedure is often appropriate for women who have had children. Surgeons reduce the breast "envelope," where there is simply too much skin holding the breast tissue. It can be done with or without using implants. There are sometimes large scars, but they can often be hidden around nipples and underneath breasts. Surgery cost averages $4,000.

Otoplasty (ear surgery)

This procedure sets prominent ears closer to the head or reduces large ears. Many doctors recommend this procedure for children, when it is sometimes covered by insurance. I consider this to be an important psychological boost to young patients, who may be the subject of ridicule during formative years. The results are permanent, and recovery time is only a week. Cost: approximately $2,500.

Eyelid Surgery (blepharoplasty)

To correct drooping upper eyelids and puffy bags below the eyes, the surgeon removes excess fat, skin, and muscle. If your vision has been impaired by the droopy lids, your insurance company often will cover a portion of this expense. The general rule of thumb is that one's visual field has to become at least 20 percent decreased for consideration by an insurance company. Recovery time is about a week.

The eyes are the portal to the soul, the most important aesthetic element of the face. A blepharoplasty can make a huge difference in your appearance and self-esteem, without looking like there was any surgery at all. Average cost: $2,500.

Face-lift (rhitidectomy)

This procedure reduces sagging skin, jowls, and loose neck skin by removing excess fat, tightening muscles, and redraping the skin. It takes several hours to complete, and a couple of weeks to recover. The results will last for as long as ten years. There are four basic surgical approaches to a face-lift:

1. A *full face-lift*, or *subcutaneous musculo-aponeurotic substance (SMAS) two-layer face-lift*, is designed to lift and tighten sagging skin, primarily in the lower two-thirds of the face. It smooths the neck, re-

duces jowls, and refines the jawline. Incisions are made behind each ear and the skin is raised. Excess fat and skin are removed, underlying tissues are repositioned, and permanent sutures hold the skin in its new position. This is the most common type of face-lift.

2. A *deep plane face-lift* lifts the facial muscles and fat under the connective tissues. This procedure goes down to the bone, allowing more facial sculpturing to correct problems in the cheeks and mid-face area, such as deep furrows between the nose and mouth. This surgery is more invasive than a full face-lift, and requires more recovery time. The effects last longer than with other face-lifts, but swelling can remain for as long as a year. There is often a scar along the hairline, and the natural hairline becomes elevated due to pulling up the skin. It is not a common procedure in the United States, and can sometimes leave the patient looking quite changed.

3. The *S-lift* is so named for the S-shaped incision made near the ear, and is sometimes called a "short scar" lift. This procedure sutures the connective tissues to the facial bones—permanently fixing the soft tissue of the cheek, for example, so it remains stable and full. This is far less invasive than a full face-lift, and is best for younger patients or those who want only minimal changes.

4. A *mid-face face-lift* is performed using tiny incisions behind the hairline and inside the mouth. Fat in the cheeks is repositioned up onto the cheekbones, which improves furrows between nose and mouth. It's the perfect surgery for deep nasolabial folds, and is sometimes called a "cheek lift."

A face-lift does not improve skin quality or droopy eyelids—other procedures must still address those conditions.

There is now a neck "sling" that reduces a saggy neck. This permanent implant is a narrow strip of Gore-Tex (which is actually a type of plastic called polytetrafluoroethylene). It is surgically attached from behind one earlobe, below the jaw and chin, up over the other earlobe. This is a newer procedure, whose long-term effects are still not known. Average cost for each type of face-lift: $5,500.

Facial Implants

This procedure changes the shape of your face or replaces lost volume by using carefully shaped implants. These are made of either silicone, Gore-Tex, or cadaver bone. They can improve a receding chin, jawline, or add cheek prominence. It takes only about an hour, and a week to recover. Scars are hidden, and the effects are often permanent, though not always. Cost: about $2,000.

Brow Lift (forehead lift)

This surgery minimizes forehead creases, and improves drooping eyebrows, hooded eyelids, and frown lines. It can refresh your appearance by "lifting" the area above the eyes. The traditional surgical technique uses an incision across the top of the head just behind the hairline. Less invasive is the endoscopic technique, which requires three or four small incisions behind the hairline. This is more commonly used today, and the scars are virtually nonexistent.

Certain muscles and tissues of the forehead are removed, to smooth out the skin. Sutures fix the revised brow tissue in place. This procedure is sometimes performed in conjunction with eyelid surgery or a face-lift. The results are quite astounding. This takes less than two hours in surgery, and lasts as long as ten years. Cost: about $3,000.

To fill in bald areas, a surgeon might reduce the skin on the scalp, or expand tissue with grafts, or, most commonly, punch grafts (plugs). This is best done on men with male pattern baldness whose hair loss has stopped. Technology has improved amazingly in recent years. We may remember the bygone man with "doll tufts." Now, doctors can place a single hair into a follicle and it is unbelievably natural in appearance. It takes up to three hours, and recovery is in five days. It may take a few months to achieve the final look of newly grown hair, but then it will be permanent. Costs start at $4,000 and escalate with size of treatment.

CO_2 Laser Resurfacing

This is a relatively invasive laser procedure using carbon dioxide to convert the light to laser. It tightens skin and eliminates wrinkles, but the burn wounds are oozing and painful throughout a lengthy recovery. I put this laser treatment in with the surgeries because I find that many patients don't understand how invasive and painful it is. I only recommend this peel for a patient who has severe "cobwebs" of wrinkles all over her face, because it involves such an arduous recovery. As I mentioned earlier, my experience shows that patients dislike this procedure more than any other. Cost: about $2,500.

Liposuction

This procedure improves body shape by using a vacuum tube to remove fat deposits that are resistant to exercise. The tumescent technique uses a saline solution to target fat cells to minimize recovery time. Common locations for liposuction are the chin, cheeks, neck, upper arms, above breasts, abdomen, buttocks, hips, thighs, knees, calves, and ankles. For large areas, an ultrasound linoplasty probe is used to liquefy the fat before it is suctioned.

This procedure is most ideal for the person who is of normal weight or only slightly overweight. It is not a quick fix for weight loss. It is for the woman who has "saddle bag" deformity or a man with pronounced "love handles," which no diet and exercise have changed.

Recovery from liposuction takes a week or two, and there is some risk of asymmetry or pigment changes. The results are only maintained through proper diet and exercise. Liposuction does not tighten skin—only skin removal or lasers can do that. Cost varies from $2,000 to $4,000.

Spot Treatments for Specific Symptoms

Age spots and wrinkles—Retin-A, hydroquinone, RéVive cream, erbium laser, medium peel

Droopy jowls—fat injection

Double chin—weight loss

Marionette lines—fat injection

Lip lines—dermabrasion, erbium laser, RéVive Sensitif or Intensité cream

Turkey gobbler—this can only be removed with surgery; it is caused by excess skin

Baggy upper eyelids—fat removal, brow lift, eyelid surgery

Veins—RéVive Sans Veines cream, laser, sclerotherapy

"Cobwebs" of facial wrinkles—CO_2 laser

Frown lines—brow lift, Botox

Dark undereye circles—RéVive Intensité Les Yeux with MPI,
    chemical or laser peel
Crow's-feet—chemical or laser peel, Botox, RéVive
Forehead lines—Botox, brow lift

All surgeries carry some serious risk, such as nerve damage, scarring, infection, or excessive bleeding. One of the greatest risks of a face-lift is that you will be disappointed with the result. You should set reasonable expectations, after detailed conversations with your plastic surgeon. Together, you can set goals and clarify expectations. Do not rely solely on computerized images to indicate the potential result. These can give you a good idea of what to expect, but they sometimes serve as a sales device to lock you in.

Be sure to research and find a qualified plastic surgeon. Many other doctors now perform cosmetic procedures, as they can be a more lucrative business than traditional medicine. In an aesthetic practice, doctors don't need to rely on insurance companies for reimbursement. Many of these doctors have no training in plastic surgery, but they are not legally prohibited from calling themselves cosmetic surgeons. Outside of a hospital, a doctor is permitted to perform any procedure he or she chooses. Board regulations do not apply to the activities inside a doctor's office. Be sure your doctor is not just "board-certified," but board-certified specifically by the American Board of Plastic Surgery (ABPS), and ideally a member of the American Society of Aesthetic Plastic Surgeons (ASAPS) whose practice is limited almost entirely to aesthetic procedures. Such doctors can be located through the Resources section in this book.

resources

How to Find a Good Skin Doctor and the Best Board-Certified Plastic Surgeon

Call or go online to find out which doctors in your area have been certified by the American Board of Plastic Surgery, a member board of the American Board of Medical Specialties (866-ASK-ABMS; www.abplsurg.org). Remember, even if a doctor is a member of the American Medical Association, he or she may not be board-certified by the ASPS.

Where to Buy Products Mentioned in This Book

Most of the products mentioned in this book can be purchased online at websites such as skinstore.com. RéVive is available at many fine stores, including Neiman Marcus, Saks Fifth Avenue, Bergdorf Goodman, and Bliss in the United States; Space.NK in the United Kingdom; Mecca in Australia; and Joyce Boutiques in Hong Kong. You can also find it online at www.reviveskincare.com and other online retailers.

WHERE TO LEARN ABOUT PENDING NEW SKIN PRODUCTS

There are great resources available at your local library or on the Internet. The *New England Journal of Medicine* and the *Journal of the American Medical Association* frequently publish articles about developing skincare technologies. These can be found online at www.NEJM.org or www. MedWebPlus.com. There are also numerous articles compiled on the website of the National Center for Biotechnical Information (NCBI) in their National Library of Medicine (also known as "Pub Med"). Check out www.NCBI.NLM.NIH.gov, or begin at www.NIH.gov and move on from there.

patent study of human
epidermal growth factor (egf)

U.S. Pat. No. 4,695,590 describes a method for retarding aging by administering synthetic chemicals, such as certain hydroxy diphenyl alkyl derivatives, preferably by oral administration. It would be desirable to avoid the internal administration of synthetic chemicals both for convenience and to avoid possible side effects of internally administered synthetic chemicals.

A variety of protein factors are known to be essential to the growth and differentiation of cells including epidermal cells. Many of these proteins extracted from tissues have been identified: such as epidermal growth factor (EGF), insulin-like growth factor (IGF), platelet-derived growth factor (PDGF), fibroblast growth factor (FGF) and the like. U.S. Pat. No. 4,959,353 describes the use of epidermal growth factor for treating corneal wounds and U.S. Pat. No. 5,130,298 describes compositions of epidermal growth factor stabilized against degradation with metal cations and used for treating wounds. U.S. Pat. No. 5,104,977 discloses use of TGF-beta with either [*sic*] TGF-alpha for treating damaged tissue. However, as these patents illustrate, protein growth factors have not been previously shown to decrease epidermal cell senescence in unabraded or nonwounded skin. It had been previously thought that large proteins such as growth factors could not penetrate uninjured or intact skin in order to reach the appropriate basal cell layers to increase cellular replication and thereby decrease epidermal cell senescence.

It would be desirable to have a simple method to decrease epidermal cell and thereby cutaneous senescence in humans with or without aesthetic and reconstructive surgery.

Summary of the Invention

The invention is directed to a method for improving the appearance of the human skin and thereby decreasing the stigmata of aging in humans by topically administering to human skin a composition comprising a mixture of protein growth factors consisting essentially of (a) epidermal growth factor (EGF) and (b) a member selected from the group consisting of transforming growth factor-alpha (TGF-α), and fibroblast growth factor (FGF) and a mixture of transforming growth factor-alpha (TGF-α) and fibroblast growth factor (FGF) in a topical cosmetically acceptable carrier, in an amount that effectively to improve [sic] the appearance of the human skin, e.g., by decreasing cutaneous senescence in humans.

It previously has been doubted that such growth factor proteins could reach the appropriate basal cell layer to produce increased cellular mitosis and hence replication. By contrast, use of the composition and method of the invention results in one or more effects such as decreased senescence of epidermal cells thereby increasing the rate of cellular replication and desquamation producing a more youthful appearance; delaying cutaneous atrophy, the thinning of epidermis and dermis and the increase of hydroxyproline content of the dermis.

DR. GREGORY BAYS BROWN has spent more than twenty years as a plastic surgeon, carefully observing the process of how skin heals. In clinical studies, he innovated the application of a human protein that actually makes skin heal faster than at its previous rate, a discovery that was originally published in the *New England Journal of Medicine*. After serving his general surgical internship and residency at Massachusetts General Hospital and the University of Louisville, Dr. Brown became a Fellow at Emory University's Division of Plastic and Reconstructive Surgery. He lives in Louisville, Kentucky, and New York City.

JANE O'BOYLE is a former publishing executive and the author of several books. She lives in Charleston, South Carolina.

about the type

This book was set in Baskerville, a typeface that was designed by John Baskerville, an amateur printer and type founder, and cut for him by John Handy in 1750. The type became popular again when the Lanston Monotype Corporation of London revised the classic Roman face in 1923. The Mergenthaler Linotype Company in England and the United States cut a version of Baskerville in 1931, making it one of the most widely used typefaces today.